Gluten-Free Sourdough Bread Recipes for Beginners

Master Healthy Baking, Create Delicious Low-Calorie, high protein Treats, and Eliminate Waste with Sourdough Discard

Samantha Bax

Gluten-Free Sourdough Bread Recipes for Beginners
Samantha Bax

Copyright 2023 © Prose Books LLC

eBook ISBN: 978-1-963160-23-9
Paperback ISBN: 978-1-963160-27-7

All rights reserved.

SKU: PBP-24103

No portion of this book may be reproduced without written permission from the publisher or author except as permitted by U.S. copyright law.

This publication is designed to provide accurate and authoritative information regarding the subject matter covered. It is sold with the understanding that neither the author nor the publisher is engaged in rendering legal, investment, accounting, or other professional services.

While the publisher and author have used their best efforts in preparing this book, they make no representations or warranties with respect to the accuracy or completeness of the contents of this book and specifically disclaim any implied warranties of merchantability or fitness for a particular purpose. Sales representatives or written sales materials may create or extend no warranty.

The advice and strategies contained herein may not be suitable for your situation. You should consult with a professional when appropriate. Neither the publisher nor the author shall be liable for any loss of profit or other commercial damages, including but not limited to special, incidental, consequential, personal, or other damages.

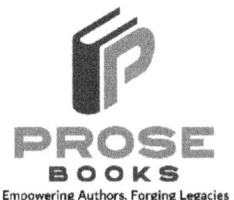

Prose Books
Prose Books LLC
Merrimack, NH 03054 USA
email: info@prosebooks.com

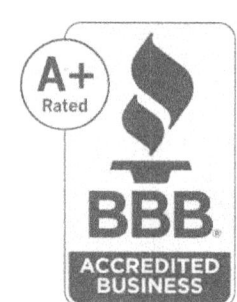

Table of Contents

Table of Contents iii
INTRODUCTION vii
Chapter 1: The Wonders of Gluten-Free Sourdough 1
Chapter 2: Tools & Ingredients for Success 3
Chapter 3: The Heart of It All – Creating Your Gluten-Free Sourdough Starter 11
Chapter 4: The Zero-Waste Kitchen: Sourdough Discard Delights 20
    Sweet Treats: Muffins (7 Recipes) 20
    Recipe #1: Tropical Chia Powerhouse 22
    Recipe #2: Sunrise Surprise Muffin 23
    Recipe #3: Almond Berry Burst 24
    Recipe #4: Chocolate Avocado Delight 25
    Recipe #5: Nutty Pear Spice 26
    Recipe #6: Savory Protein Kick 27
    Recipe #7: Raspberry & Quinoa Power 28
Chapter 5: Pancakes & Waffles (6 Recipes) 29
    Recipe 8: Protein-Packed Pumpkin Power 31
    Recipe 9: Fluffy Banana & Greek Yogurt 32
    Recipe 10: Kiwi Chia Burst 33
    Recipe 11: Jackfruit & Coconut Surprise 34
    Recipe 12: Carrot Cake Fusion 35
    Recipe 13: Savory Ricotta & Herb 36
Chapter 6: Bread Pudding (4 Recipes) 37
    Recipe 14: Spiced Pear Delight 39
    Recipe 15: Tropical Twist 40
    Recipe 16: Berry Burst 41
    Recipe 17: Chocolate & Cherry Indulgence 42
Chapter 7: Cookies (8 Recipes) 43
    Recipe 18: Oatmeal Apricot Power 45
    Recipe 19: Nutty Chocolate Chip 46
    Recipe 20: Pumpkin Seed & Spice 47
    Recipe 21: Banana Chia Bites 48
    Recipe 22: PB & J Swirl 49
    Recipe 23: Blueberry Lemon Zest 50
    Recipe 24: Tropical Coconut Bites 51

- Recipe 25: Tropical Coconut Bites 52
- Recipe 26: Double Chocolate Delight 53

Chapter 8: Savory Sensations: Crackers & Crostini (7 Recipes) 54
- Recipe 27: Seeded Powerhouse Crackers 56
- Recipe 28: Chickpea & Herb Surprise 57
- Recipe 29: Zesty Parmesan & Almond 58
- Recipe 30: Spiced Lentil & Quinoa 59
- Recipe 31: Everything Bagel Crostini 60
- Recipe 32: Smoky Paprika & Chickpea 61
- Recipe 33: Mediterranean Olive & Feta Crumble 62

Chapter 9: Breadcrumbs (5 Recipes + Uses) 63
- Recipe 34: Classic Herbed Breadcrumbs 64
- Recipe 35: Protein-Packed Breadcrumbs 65
- Recipe 36: Spiced Panko-Style 66
- Recipe 37: Quinoa & Almond Crumbs 67
- Recipe 38: Lemony Herb Breadcrumbs 68

Chapter 10: Stuffing & Panzanella (6 Recipes) 69
- Recipe 39: Quinoa, Kale & Cranberry 71
- Recipe 40: Mediterranean Panzanella 72
- Recipe 41: Southwestern Black Bean & Corn 73
- Recipe 42: Lentil & Mushroom Stuffing 74
- Recipe 43: Sausage & Apple Delight 75
- Recipe 44: Greek-Inspired Panzanella 76

Chapter 11: Pretzels (7 recipes) 77
- Recipe 45: Classic Soft Pretzels 79
- Recipe 46: Cheesy Jalapeño Pretzel Bites 80
- Recipe 47: Cinnamon Sugar Pretzel Twists 81
- Recipe 48: Ham & Cheese Stuffed Pretzels 82
- Recipe 49: Spiced Pumpkin Pretzel Knots 83
- Recipe 50: Everything Bagel Pretzels 84
- Recipe 51: Herbed Garlic Pretzel Sticks 85

Chapter 12: Beyond the Bread: Sourdough Adventures Sourdough Pizza Crust (5 Recipes) 86
- Recipe 52: Mediterranean Feast Pizza 87
- Recipe 53: Thai-Inspired Chicken Pizza 88
- Recipe 54: Lentil & Veggie Lover's Pizza 89
- Recipe 55: Shrimp & Avocado Delight 90
- Recipe 56: Spicy Chorizo & Pineapple 91

Chapter 13: Sourdough Bagels (5 Recipes) 92
- Recipe 57: Protein Power Bagel 94
- Recipe 58: Spiced Lentil & Quinoa 95

- Recipe 59: "Everything" Meets Sourdough 96
- Recipe 60: Blueberry Almond Swirl 97
- Recipe 61: Sundried Tomato & Olive 98

Chapter 14: Sourdough Cinnamon Rolls (5 Recipes) 99
- Recipe 62: High-Protein Cinnamon Rolls 101
- Recipe 63: Pumpkin Spice Swirl 102
- Recipe 64: Apple Walnut Delight 103
- Recipe 65: Tropical Twist 104
- Recipe 66: Chocolate & Cherry Indulgence 105

Chapter 15: Sourdough Biscuits (5 Recipes) 106
- Recipe 67: Chicken & Herb Biscuits 108
- Recipe 68: Ham & Cheddar Drop Biscuits 109
- Recipe 69: Sweet Potato & Pecan (Gluten-Free) 110
- Recipe 70: Spiced Carrot & Raisin Biscuits (Gluten-Free) 111
- Recipe 71: Pumpkin Seed & Cranberry Delight (Gluten-Free) 112

Chapter 16: Creative Leftover Uses (5 Recipes) 113
- Recipe 72: French Toast Extravaganza 115
- Recipe 73: Gourmet Grilled Cheese 116
- Recipe 74: Panzanella Powerhouse 117
- Recipe 75: Sourdough Bread Pudding 118
- Recipe 76: Savory Croutons 119

Chapter 17: Advanced Techniques & Flavor Exploration 120

Chapter 18: Accompaniments for Your Sourdough 126
- Recipe 77: Quinoa & Avocado Hummus 128
- Recipe 78: Roasted Red Pepper & Feta Dip 129
- Recipe 79: White Bean & Spinach Spread 130
- Recipe 80: Sundried Tomato & Basil Pesto 131
- Recipe 81: Lentil & Carrot Dip 132
- Recipe 82: Smoked Paprika & Cashew Cheese 133

Chapter 19: Soups & Stews to Pair with Sourdough (6 Recipes) 134
- Recipe 83: Creamy Carrot & Quinoa Soup 136
- Recipe 84: Hearty Lentil & Kale Stew 137
- Recipe 85: Tomato & White Bean Bisque 138
- Recipe 86: Spiced Butternut Squash & Chickpea Soup 139
- Recipe 87: Creamy Asparagus & Spinach Soup 140
- Recipe 88: Classic Gazpacho: Revitalized 141

Chapter 20: Salad Dressings Enhanced by Sourdough Crumbs (6 Recipes) 142
- Recipe 89: Creamy Herb & Sourdough Crumb Vinaigrette 144
- Recipe 90: Roasted Garlic & Parmesan Vinaigrette 145
- Recipe 91: Tahini, Lemon & Sourdough Crumb Dressing 146

- Recipe 92: Spiced Carrot & Ginger Dressing 147
- Recipe 93: Avocado & Lime Vinaigrette 148
- Recipe 94: Balsamic & Berry Vinaigrette 149

Chapter 21: Creative Sourdough Crumb Uses (7 Recipes) 150
- Recipe 95: Herb-Crusted Fish 151
- Recipe 96: Quinoa & Sourdough Stuffed Peppers 152
- Recipe 97: Roasted Vegetable Gratin 153
- Recipe 98: Roasted Cauliflower Steaks 154
- Recipe 99: Baked Mac & Cheese Topping 155
- Recipe 100: Savory Breakfast Crumble 156
- Recipe 101 Fruit & Sourdough Crumble 157

Chapter 22: Nutritional Notes and Recipe Adaptations 158

Meal Plan Structure 161

About The Author 167

Other Books By Samantha Bax 169

Thank You 172

BONUS: FREE Meal-Planner 173

INTRODUCTION

Introduction to Gluten-Free Sourdough Bread Recipes for Beginners

Welcome to *"Gluten-Free Sourdough Bread Recipes for Beginners,"* your essential guide to mastering the art of gluten-free sourdough baking. This book is designed for anyone looking to dive into the world of gluten-free baking without sacrificing flavor, texture, or the joy of creating beautiful, homemade bread. Whether you're a novice baker or someone with dietary restrictions eager to indulge in sourdough's unique tang and chewy texture, this book is your perfect companion.

Within these pages, you'll discover how to harness the natural power of a gluten-free sourdough starter, a living ingredient that imparts depth and complexity to your bread. This guide is structured to take you from the basics of maintaining a healthy starter to crafting a variety of bread and other baked goods, all while keeping your creations low-calorie and high in protein.

Here's What You'll Learn:

- **The Basics of Gluten-Free Sourdough:** Understand the fundamentals of sourdough baking, including how to cultivate and maintain a gluten-free sourdough starter. You'll learn why sourdough is a superior choice for health-conscious bakers and how its natural fermentation process can benefit those sensitive to gluten.
- **Healthy Baking Techniques:** Explore alternative flours and natural ingredients that don't just mimic traditional flavors but enhance them. From brown rice flour to almond flour, discover how these gluten-free alternatives can be used to make delicious sourdough bread.
- **Delicious, Nutritious Recipes:** Each recipe is crafted to maximize flavor without gluten. Enjoy a variety of bread, from classic boules to flavorful focaccias, alongside creative ways to use sourdough discard in pancakes, muffins, and more, ensuring you produce zero waste.
- **Low-Calorie, High-Protein Options:** Focus on recipes that cater to a health-conscious lifestyle, with detailed nutritional information provided for each creation. Whether you're looking to build muscle, lose weight, or eat healthier, these recipes are designed to align with your fitness and health goals.
- **Practical Tips and Tricks:** Gain valuable insights into gluten-free sourdough baking, including troubleshooting common issues, understanding hydration levels in gluten-free flours, and learning how to achieve the perfect crust and crumb every time.

"Gluten-Free Sourdough Bread Recipes for Beginners" is more than just a cookbook—it's a journey into the heart of artisan baking without gluten. Whether you're baking for health reasons or love the process, this book will provide all the tools you need to succeed. Embrace the challenge and delight of gluten-free sourdough baking and transform the way you cook and eat, one delicious loaf at a time. Join us as we break bread in the most nutritious and flavorful way possible and let your baking adventure begin!

Gluten-Free Sourdough Bread Recipes for Beginners - Samantha Bax

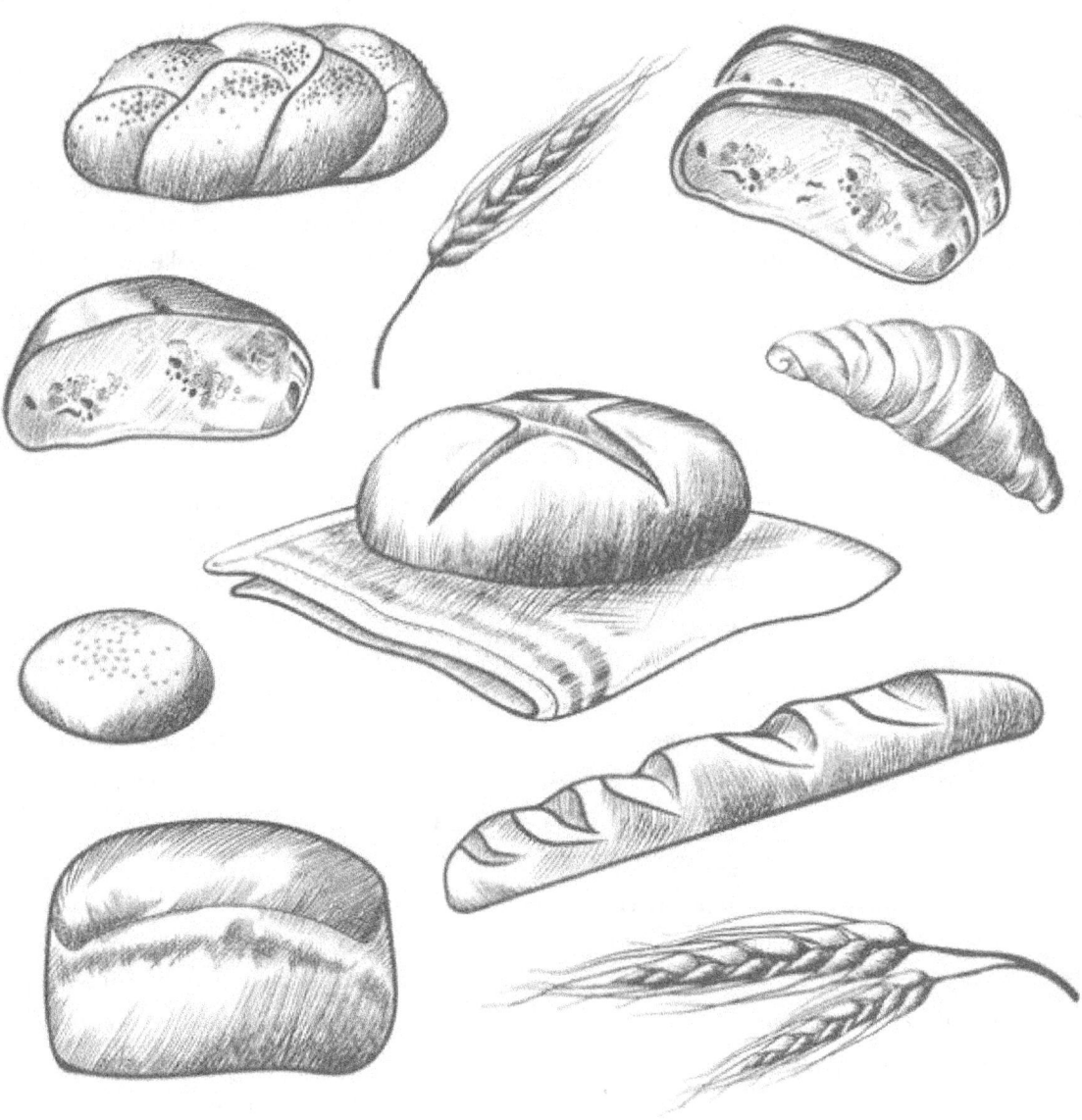

Chapter 1: The Wonders of Gluten-Free Sourdough

Forget Everything You Think You Know About Gluten-Free Bread

Look, I get it. Gluten-free bread has a reputation, and let's be honest – it isn't always a good one. Dense, crumbly, gummy...we've all been there. But hear me out: sourdough changes EVERYTHING. This isn't your grocery store gluten-free loaf. This is a whole new world of flavor, texture, and downright good eating'.

Why Sourdough? The Magic of Fermentation

Sourdough isn't just about ditching the gluten; it's about embracing good-for-you bacteria and the wild yeast that's all around us. See those little critters in your starter? They're the real heroes. They break down those tough gluten-free starches, making your bread easier to digest.

But wait, there's more! The magic of fermentation adds this incredible depth of flavor – a subtle tang, a hint of something special that regular bread can't touch.

Your Starter: The Heart of Your Sourdough Journey

Think of your starter as your kitchen pet. Quirky, a bit high-maintenance, but oh-so-worth it. It's a living thing, a bubbling, breathing testament to the wonders of nature and a little bit of your kitchen magic.

Please don't be scared; I'll take you by the hand. We'll cover the following:

- **Types of Gluten-Free Flours:** Because your starter needs good food! We'll explore the best options and how they create different textures.
- **The Art of Feeding:** How to keep your little beastie happy, healthy, and ready to make your bread rise.

- **Troubleshooting 101:** Hooch? Sluggish starter? No worries, we'll tackle those common hiccups together.
- **Shaping Beautiful Loaves:** Master the art of perfectly scored batards, stunning boules, and intricate braids.
- **Whole Grain & Seed Power:** Incorporate spelt, rye, oats, sunflower seeds, pumpkin seeds, and more - boosting flavor and nutrition.
- **Naturally Sweetened:** Discover hints of sweetness without the sugar rush, using fruits, spices, and the secret power of malt.
- **Seasonal Inspiration:** Tap into the bounty of each season – from spring's herbs and berries to winter's citrus and spices.
- **Creative Recipes Galore:** Explore a treasure trove of recipes, including everything from protein-packed muffins, savory crackers, and showstopper pizzas to decadent bread puddings and festive holiday bakes.

Buckle up, bakers, because this gluten-free sourdough adventure is about to get wild and delicious!

Chapter 2: Tools & Ingredients for Success

Starting your baking journey, especially when delving into the realm of sourdough, requires more than excitement; it calls for the tools and ingredients. In this section, our focus is on providing you with all the elements to make sure your sourdough baking is not only successful but also enjoyable.

The key to baking begins with understanding and choosing top-notch ingredients. We'll begin by looking into the kinds of flour that work best for sourdough, including variations that can impact the taste, texture, and rise of your bread. Flour, water, salt, and your starter are other elements. We'll talk about how the quality of each can significantly affect your end product.

Yet being a baker isn't about having ingredients—having the right tools is essential, too. This section will outline the equipment that every sourdough baker should have in their kitchen. From mixing bowls to proofing baskets Dutch ovens to baking stones, each tool plays a role in the art of sourdough baking. We'll offer suggestions on what to consider when choosing these items so that you pick tools that improve your efficiency and effectiveness in baking.

Moreover, we will explore the known yet vital tools, like dough scrapers, digital scales, and thermometers, that play a crucial role in achieving accuracy and consistency in your baking projects. Mastering the use of these accessories will enhance your baking skills. Empower you to experiment and perfect your techniques.

At the conclusion of this section, you'll be fully equipped with a stocked kitchen containing all the ingredients and tools. This readiness will pave the way for you to immerse yourself in the gratifying art of sourdough baking, armed with both knowledge and equipment to produce bread every time. Let's ensure that your baking setup matches your enthusiasm for sourdough!

Must-Have Baking Tools (and Substitutes)

Embarking on your free sourdough adventure requires essential tools, but fret not, as most of them are likely already present in your kitchen! Here's a breakdown of the items and some innovative alternatives.

Must-Have Tools:

- **Large Mixing Bowls (Glass or Non-Reactive Materials):** Why? These bowls are perfect for mixing your starter and dough. Glass or non-reactive materials (like stainless steel) won't absorb odors or alter the flavor of your starter. They also allow you to easily monitor the consistency of your starter as it ferments.

- **Alternatives:** If you don't have large bowls, a large pot or even a clean, food-grade plastic container can work in a pinch.

- **Clean Jar for Your Starter (with Loose-Fitting Lid):** Why? A dedicated jar is your starter's home! It provides a clean environment for fermentation and allows gas to escape through the loose lid. Glass jars are ideal because you can easily see the activity of your starter.

- **Alternatives:** Any clean, airtight container can work. An unused food container or even a clean, empty coffee mug can suffice. Just remember to loosen the lid slightly to allow gas to escape.

- **Spatulas and Dough Scrapers:** Why? These tools are your helping hands when mixing your starter and dough. Spatulas help fold and scrape down the sides of your container, ensuring everything gets incorporated. Dough scrapers are handy for cleaning your work surface and dividing dough.

- **Alternatives:** A spoon can replace a spatula in a pinch. A butter knife or even a clean credit card can be used as a makeshift dough scraper.

- **Digital Kitchen Scale (for Precision):** Why? Baking, especially gluten-free baking, benefits greatly from precision. A digital scale ensures accurate measurements of your flour and other ingredients, leading to consistent starter and bread results.

- **Alternatives:** While a scale is ideal, you can use measuring cups if necessary. However, keep in mind that scooping flour can compact it, leading to inaccurate measurements. If using cups, gently spoon in your flour and level it off with the back of a knife for better accuracy.

Nice-to-Have Tools:

- **Proofing Basket:** Why? A proofing basket, typically made of cane or banneton, helps shape and support your dough as it rises. It creates a beautiful textured surface on your bread and provides a controlled environment for proofing.
- **Alternatives:** While a proofing basket offers some advantages, you can still achieve good results without one. A clean, floured kitchen towel or even a colander lined with a cloth can be used for proofing.
- **Baking Stone or Dutch Oven:** Why? These baking tools help create a steamy environment in your oven, mimicking a professional bakery's steam injection. This steam is crucial for good oven rise in gluten-free sourdough bread.
- **Alternatives:** A preheated baking sheet with a shallow pan of water placed on the bottom rack of your oven can create a similar steam effect, although the results might not be identical to a baking stone or Dutch oven.
- **Lame or Sharp Knife (for Scoring Loaves):** Why? Scoring the top of your dough before baking allows controlled expansion and prevents your bread from cracking unevenly. A lame is a specialized tool with a razor blade designed for scoring, but a sharp knife can also work.
- **Alternatives:** If you don't have a lame or sharp enough knife, you can try gently scoring the top of your dough with wet fingertips.

Gluten-Free Flours: A Comprehensive Guide - Unveiling the Powerhouse Blends

In the world of gluten-free sourdough, flour becomes the building blocks of your delicious and healthy bread. The following are some fantastic options, along with their unique properties and nutritional benefits:

Brown Rice Flour:

- **The Backbone:** This mild-flavored flour is a staple in many gluten-free sourdough blends due to its neutral taste and ability to absorb moisture. It provides a good foundation for structure.
- **Nutrition:** Brown rice flour is a good source of carbohydrates for energy but is lower in protein compared to some other options. It's also a decent source of fiber.
- **Tips:** Brown rice flour can be slightly gritty, so blending it with other flour can improve texture. Look for varieties labeled "fine grind" for a smoother texture in your starter.

Millet Flour:

- **Sweet Touch:** This sweet flour brings flavor to your sourdough creations, blending well with other flours for a harmonious taste.

- **Nutritional Value:** Millet flour offers a greater amount of carbs and protein than other gluten-free options packed with iron and essential minerals.
- **Tips:** Since millet flour can be dense, it is best used in moderation or mixed with lighter flour, like brown rice. Experiment to discover the balance!

Buckwheat Flour:

- **Flavor:** Buckwheat flour provides an earthy taste that adds depth to your sourdough bread. Use it sparingly to avoid overpowering the flavor profile.
- **Nutrition Facts:** Buckwheat flour is a protein source containing all amino acids (a rarity among plant-based proteins) along with fiber and B vitamins.
- **Tips:** To balance its heaviness, pair buckwheat flour with lighter options strategically for enhanced flavor without compromising texture.

Sorghum Flour:

- **Light & Mild:** Sorghum flour is a choice for giving structure to your sourdough bread without imparting a taste. The subtle flavor of sorghum flour allows the true essence of the ingredients to stand out.
- **Nutritional Value:** Sorghum flour is rich in carbohydrates and fiber and has a protein content that is higher than that of other gluten-free alternatives.
- **Cooking Tip:** To achieve a lighter texture, mix sorghum flour with lighter flour. It has moisture absorption, so adjust your measurements accordingly.

Exploring Other Flour Varieties like Amaranth, Teff, Quinoa, and Gluten Free Oat Flour

- **Amaranth Flour:** Delicately nutty with a hint of lightness, it offers protein and fiber content.
- **Teff Flour:** Earthy and slightly sweet teff brings depth to dishes and is packed with calcium and iron.
- **Quinoa Flour:** While slightly bitter, on its own, quinoa flour contributes well to blends and provides protein.

- **Gluten-Free Oat Flour:** Imparts tenderness and a subtle sweetness; make sure it's certified gluten-free if you have the disease. The Power of Blending:

Now that you've met some incredible flours remember that magic happens in the blend! Combining different flours creates a synergy that enhances the overall texture, flavor, and nutrition of your sourdough bread. Experiment with combinations of these flours to find your perfect balance!

Tips:

- ✓ **Freshness Matters:** Choose flours with recent milling dates for optimal performance in your starter and bread.
- ✓ **Fine vs. Coarse Grinds:** Finer grinds are generally preferred for creating a smooth starter. You can adjust the grind size depending on the texture of the final bread.
- ✓ **Storage:** Store your flour in airtight containers in a cool, dry place to maintain freshness.

Starches, Binders, & Beyond: Mastering Texture & Rise

While gluten-free flour provides the foundation for your sourdough, certain ingredients play a supporting role in mimicking the structure and texture that gluten usually provides.

1. Psyllium Husk: The Star Performer

- **What it is:** Psyllium husk comes from the seeds of the Plantago ovata plant. When combined with water, it forms a thick, gel-like substance.
- **How it helps:** This gel imitates gluten's binding power, helping trap gas bubbles and improving the rise and texture of your sourdough bread. It also adds moisture, preventing your dough from drying out.
- **Nutrition:** Psyllium husk is an excellent source of soluble fiber, promoting gut health and regularity.
- **Tips:** A little psyllium husk goes a long way! Start with 1-2 teaspoons per cup of gluten-free flour in your starter and bread recipes.

2. Xanthan Gum: The Versatile Assistant

- **What it is:** A naturally derived gum produced by bacteria fermentation, commonly added to gluten-free baked goods.

- **How it helps:** Like psyllium husk, xanthan gum acts as a binder, enhancing the texture and preventing crumbliness, but in smaller quantities. It also adds elasticity to your dough, improving its ability to hold its shape.
- **Nutrition:** Xanthan gum is a soluble fiber but offers less nutritional benefit than psyllium husk.
- **Tips:** Use xanthan gum sparingly. Start with 1/4 teaspoon per cup of gluten-free flour and increase slightly if needed. Too much can make your bread gummy.

3. The Supporting Cast: Tapioca Starch & Potato Starch

- **What they are:** These neutral-flavored starches are derived from tapioca and potato tubers, respectively.
- **How they help:** Starches add tenderness and a light, slightly chewy texture to your sourdough bread. They also help with moisture retention and improve overall structure.
- **Nutrition:** Starches are primarily carbohydrates and offer fewer nutritional benefits than psyllium husk.
- **Tips:** Incorporate a small amount of starch (approximately 1-2 tablespoons per cup of gluten-free flour) in your recipes. Too much can create a dense and overly chewy loaf.

The Art of Combining

Just like with gluten-free flours, experimenting with these ingredients in various combinations will help you achieve the perfect texture profile for your sourdough creations. Here's a starting point:

- **Basic Blend:** Psyllium husk (or a combination of psyllium husk and xanthan gum), along with a small amount of starch, makes a versatile base for many recipes.
- **Experimentation Encouraged:** Try incorporating small amounts of other gluten-free starches (like arrowroot or corn starch) for unique results.

Additional Considerations

- **Hydration Matters:** Starches and binders absorb water. Adjust your recipe's hydration levels accordingly to avoid dough that is too dry.
- **Whole vs. Powdered:** You can use either whole psyllium husk or its powdered form. If using whole husk, grind it finer for better incorporation into your starter.

Sweeteners, Fats & Flavorings: Unveiling the Delicious & Nutritious

In gluten-free sourdough, we not only focus on creating amazing texture but also cater to a variety of dietary needs and flavor preferences. Let's explore the world of sweeteners, fats, and flavorings that will elevate your baking experience!

Sweeteners: Beyond the Basics

Sugar feeds the wild yeast in your starter, but when it comes to sweetening your bread, a variety of options exist, especially for those with special dietary needs:

- **Natural Sweeteners:**
    - **Honey:** A classic choice, honey offers a subtle floral sweetness and provides some beneficial nutrients like antioxidants. However, it's not suitable for vegans.
    - **Maple Syrup:** This natural sweetener boasts a deeper, richer flavor than honey and is a good source of minerals like manganese and zinc.
    - **Molasses:** A darker option with a robust flavor, molasses adds depth and moisture to your bread. It's a good source of iron and other minerals but be mindful of its higher sugar content. (Note: While these sweeteners feed the starter, using less refined options aligns with a focus on healthier choices.)

- **Special Dietary Considerations:**

    - **Sugar Alcohols (Erythritol, Xylitol):** These sugar alcohols provide sweetness without significantly impacting blood sugar levels. However, use them in moderation, as excessive intake can cause digestive issues.
    - **Monk Fruit Sweetener:** This natural sweetener derived from a Chinese gourd is a great option for those seeking a very low-carb sweetener.

    - **Tips:** Experiment with different sweeteners to find your preference. Start with a smaller amount and adjust to taste, remembering that some sweeteners are naturally sweeter than others.

Fats: Adding Richness (Use Sparingly)

While fat isn't essential in gluten-free sourdough, a small amount can enhance the flavor and texture of your bread:

- **Olive Oil:** A healthy source of monounsaturated fats, olive oil adds a subtle flavor and improves crumb texture. Use a light variety to avoid overpowering the taste.
- **Melted Butter:** For a richer flavor, a small amount of melted butter can be incorporated. However, be mindful that butter can affect the rise of your bread.

Flavor Boosters: Unleash Your Creativity!

This is where your sourdough journey gets truly exciting! Explore a world of flavor possibilities with:

- **Herbs:** Rosemary, thyme, and oregano add a savory touch perfect for sandwich bread.
- **Spices:** Cinnamon, nutmeg, and ginger add warmth and sweetness, which is ideal for breakfast loaves.
- **Seeds:** Sunflower, pumpkin, and chia seeds add a delightful crunch and texture.
- **Extracts:** Almond, vanilla, and orange extracts offer subtle flavor nuances.

Experimentation is Key!

Don't be afraid to combine different flavorings to create unique sourdough masterpieces. Here are some starting points:

- **Savory:** Rosemary and olive oil
- **Sweet:** Cinnamon, raisins, and walnuts
- **Fruity:** Orange zest and cranberries

Remember, successful baking is about balance. Start with subtle additions of flavorings and adjust to your taste preferences.

***Maintain a Consistent Feeding Schedule**: "Keep your sourdough starter healthy by feeding it regularly at the same time each day to ensure consistent activity and readiness for baking."*

Chapter 3: The Heart of It All – Creating Your Gluten-Free Sourdough Starter

Embarking on the journey of gluten-free sourdough baking begins with one crucial element: the sourdough starter. This chapter is dedicated to guiding you through the process of creating and maintaining a gluten-free sourdough starter, the very heart of all your gluten-free sourdough recipes. A healthy, active starter is key to achieving delicious, well-risen breads without the use of traditional wheat flour.

Crafting your gluten-free sourdough starter involves nurturing a mixture of gluten-free flour and water, allowing it to ferment naturally. This process captures wild yeast from the environment and beneficial bacteria that ferment the dough, imparting the classic sourdough tang and leavening the bread naturally. We will explore various gluten-free flours—such as rice, sorghum, and buckwheat—that can be used to initiate and sustain your starter, each offering unique flavors and benefits.

This chapter will not only teach you how to start your gluten-free sourdough culture but also how to care for it daily. You'll learn the signs of a healthy starter and how to troubleshoot common issues such as lack of activity or unwanted mold. Regular feeding, understanding the starter's environment, and knowing how to use it in recipes are all part of the journey.

Additionally, we will delve into the science behind a gluten-free sourdough starter, discussing how the fermentation process works and why it is beneficial for those with gluten sensitivities. The goal is to empower you with the knowledge and skills to create a vibrant starter that will serve as the foundation for all your gluten-free baking adventures.

Get ready to embrace the art of gluten-free sourdough baking. With your new starter, you'll be able to produce breads that are not only safe for those with gluten intolerance but are also deliciously rich in flavor and perfect in texture. Let's begin this transformative process, bringing the magic of sourdough into a gluten-free kitchen.

Understanding the Power of a Sourdough Starter

Before I go into recipes, here's a quick recap on why this bubbly, alive mixture is so important:

- **Natural Rise:** Wild yeast and bacteria in your starter give your bread lift without needing commercial yeast.
- **Unique Flavor:** A sourdough starter adds a delicious, slightly tangy flavor that sets your bread apart from store-bought varieties.

- **Improved Gut Health:** The fermentation process in sourdough can make it easier to digest and potentially more nutritious.

Mastering the Basic Loaf

Simple Gluten-Free Sourdough (Step-by-Step Guide)

Ingredients:

- Active gluten-free sourdough starter (e.g., your brown rice starter)
- Gluten-free flour blend (start with brown rice, tapioca starch, millet flour)
- Psyllium husk powder
- Water (filtered is best)
- Salt
- (Optional) A touch of honey or maple syrup
- (Optional) A small amount of olive oil

Equipment:

- Large mixing bowl
- Kitchen scale
- Baking sheet or loaf pan
- Dutch oven or baking stone (optional but recommended)

Instructions

1. **Feeding:** Ensure your starter is bubbly and active. Feed it a few hours before making your dough.

2. **Mix Dry Ingredients:** Combine your gluten-free flours, psyllium husk powder, and salt in a large mixing bowl.

3. **Activate the Starter:** In a separate bowl, combine a portion of your active starter with warm water and a touch of natural sweetener (if using). Let it sit for a few minutes to become frothy.

4. **Combine:** Add the activated starter mixture and olive oil (if using) to the dry ingredients. Mix until a shaggy dough forms.

5. **Rise:** Cover the bowl loosely and let it rise in a warm place for several hours until it increases in size (exact time depends on starter strength and temperature).

6. **Shape:** Gently shape your dough into a loaf or boule (round shape). Place it on a parchment-lined baking sheet or in a well-greased loaf pan.

7. **Final Rise:** Cover and let it rise again for 1-2 hours or until it has slightly puffed up.

8. **Score:** Lightly slash the top of the loaf with a sharp knife or lame for controlled expansion.

9. **Bake:** Preheat your oven to 450°F (232°C). If using a Dutch oven, preheat it as well. Bake for 30 minutes, then reduce heat to 400°F (204°C) and bake for another 15-20 minutes, or until the internal temperature reaches 205-210°F (96-99°C).

10. **Cool:** Let the bread cool completely on a wire rack before slicing.

Flavorful Variations

- **Seeds:** Add sunflower seeds, pumpkin seeds, or chia seeds for texture and nutrients.
- **Dried Fruit:** Cranberries, raisins, or chopped dried apricots create a sweet and fruity loaf.
- **Herbs & Spices:** Explore savory combinations like rosemary & sea salt or cinnamon & ginger.

Troubleshooting Common Issues

- **Dense Loaf:** Try increasing the psyllium husk slightly or adding a bit of xanthan gum. Ensure your starter is very active.
- **Pale Crust:** Start with a hotter initial bake temperature or brush the loaf with a light egg wash before baking.
- **Gummy Texture:** Reduce the amount of psyllium husk or try a different gluten-free flour blend.

Tips

- **Hydration:** Gluten-free sourdough doughs often need higher hydration (more water) than traditional wheat-based ones.
- **Patience:** Rising times can vary. Focus on visual cues (the dough should look larger and slightly puffy) before proceeding.

***Measure Ingredients by Weight**: "Always weigh your ingredients, especially flour and water, to achieve consistent and reliable sourdough bread results."*

Sourdough Starter Recipe #1: Basic Brown Rice Starter

- **Ingredients:**

- Brown rice flour (finely ground)
- Filtered water (chlorine-free is best)

Why These Ingredients: Brown rice flour is an accessible and neutral-tasting base, ideal for beginners. Filtered water ensures no chlorine interacts with the starter's development.

- **Step-by-Step Instructions**

1. **Day 1 (Initial Creation):** In a clean jar, combine 50 grams of brown rice flour and 50 grams of filtered water. Stir until completely mixed (it'll resemble thick pancake batter). Cover loosely with a lid or cheesecloth. Place in a warm location (around 75-80°F / 24-27°C if possible).

2. **Days 2-7 (Feeding):** Once daily, discard about half the starter. Add 50 grams of brown rice flour and 50 grams of filtered water, stirring thoroughly. Cover loosely.

3. **Signs of Life:** Look for bubbles on the surface, a slightly sour/yeasty aroma, and the starter increasing in volume before falling back (indicating it's active and hungry for feeding).

4. **Ready to Bake?** Typically, within 5-7 days, your starter should be bubbly and doubling in size before needing a feeding. This signifies it's strong enough to bake with, but the flavor will continue to develop over time.

Troubleshooting

- **No Activity:** If it's slow to start, check the temperature (too cold can slow things down). Ensure your ingredients are fresh.
- **Smells Bad:** Unpleasant odors could signify unwanted bacteria. If it seems off, it's best to start fresh with a new jar and clean utensils.

Sourdough Starter Recipe #2: Millet & Buckwheat Blend Starter

Ingredients:

- Millet flour
- Buckwheat flour
- Filtered water.

Why This Blend: Millet brings sweetness, and buckwheat adds a robust, earthy flavor profile.

- **Instructions:** Follow the same feeding schedule and process as the Basic Brown Rice Starter, using a 50/50 ratio of millet flour to buckwheat flour for your feedings.

Experimentation Encouraged!

- **The Basic Ratio:** A good starting point is 1 part flour to 1 part water by weight. Adjust the consistency as needed (thicker or thinner) based on your preference.
- **Try Your Favorites:** Experiment with different gluten-free flours like sorghum, teff, or quinoa.

Additional Tips

- ✓ **Consistency Matters:** A slightly runny batter is ideal. Think pancake batter, not thick dough.
- ✓ **Jar Size:** Start with a small jar; as the starter grows, you can upgrade to a larger one.
- ✓ **Mark the Levels:** A rubber band around the jar helps track the starter's growth.

2. Sorghum Flour: The Light & Versatile Choice

- **Characteristics:** Sorghum flour has a mild, neutral flavor that won't overpower other ingredients in your sourdough. It's light in color and texture, contributing to a good rise and tender crumb.
- **Nutrition Boost:** Sorghum is a powerhouse of protein and fiber compared to many other gluten-free options. It's also a good source of iron and other minerals.
- **Best Uses:** Sorghum works beautifully in blends, adding structure and a subtle sweetness to your bread. Pair it with other gluten-free flours like brown rice and tapioca starch for a balanced loaf.

Variations to Try

- **Classic Sandwich Loaf:** Combine sorghum flour with brown rice flour, psyllium husk, and a touch of tapioca starch for a light and sturdy loaf perfect for slicing. Add herbs like rosemary and thyme for a savory twist.
- **Fruity Breakfast Bread:** Blend sorghum with a smaller amount of brown rice flour and a touch of buckwheat for subtle depth. Add warm spices like cinnamon and ginger, plus dried cranberries, or raisins for a sweet and satisfying breakfast treat.

3. Amaranth: The Ancient Grain with a Unique Touch

- **Characteristics:** Amaranth imparts a subtle nutty and earthy flavor to your sourdough, adding a delightful complexity. It's naturally slightly sticky, which can aid in binding your dough together.
- **Nutritional Powerhouse:** This ancient grain is an excellent source of protein, fiber, iron, and calcium. Its nutritional profile makes it a valuable addition to your gluten-free baking.
- **Best Uses:** Amaranth works best in small amounts within a balanced gluten-free flour blend. It provides a unique depth of flavor and enhanced nutrition.

Variations to Try

- **Seeded Celebration Loaf**: Combine amaranth with brown rice, millet, and psyllium husk. Add a generous mix of sunflower seeds, pumpkin seeds, and chia seeds for a hearty and flavorful bread perfect for toasting.
- **Subtly Sweet & Nutty:** Blend amaranth with teff flour, a touch of sorghum, and psyllium husk for a slightly sweet and complex flavor profile. Fold in chopped walnuts or pecans for an extra touch of richness.

Important Notes:

- **Freshness Matters:** Always use fresh amaranth flour, as it can develop a bitter taste when rancid.
- **Experimentation is Key:** Start with smaller proportions of amaranth in your blends and gradually increase it as you become familiar with its unique properties.

Where to Find Them: Sorghum and amaranth flour are often found in well-stocked supermarkets, health food stores, or online.

General Sourdough Starter Guidelines

Remember, the basic process remains the same regardless of your chosen flour:

- **Initial Mix:** Combine equal parts flour and filtered water (by weight) for a thick, pancake batter-like consistency.
- **Daily Feeding:** Discard about half the starter. Replenish with equal parts flour and water.
- **Environment:** Keep your starter in a warm place (around 75-80°F / 24-27°C) and loosely covered.
- **Signs of Life:** Look for bubbles, a slightly sour smell, and rise and fall, indicating your starter is hungry and active.

Sorghum Sourdough Starter

1. **Day 1:** In a clean jar, mix 50g sorghum flour with 50g filtered water. Stir well.

2. **Days 2-7:** Feed once a day. Discard half the starter, then add 50g sorghum flour and 50g water.

3. **Why Sorghum?:** Its neutral flavor makes it a versatile base for your starter. Sorghum provides structure due to its protein content, encouraging a good rise.

Amaranth Sourdough Starter

1. **Day 1:** In a clean jar, combine 50g amaranth flour with 50g filtered water. Stir well.

2. **Days 2-7:** Follow the same daily feeding as the sorghum starter: discard half, then add 50g amaranth flour and 50g water.

3. **Why Amaranth?** Amaranth adds a subtle nutty flavor and boosts the nutritional profile of your starter. Its slight stickiness can help with binding your dough later on.

Tips for Success

- **Blended Starters:** Consider combining sorghum or amaranth with brown rice flour (50/50 ratio) for a balanced starter with good rise and a less pronounced amaranth flavor.
- **Activity Monitoring:** The exact time to achieve a mature starter varies. Focus on visual cues: doubling in size, a bubbly surface, and a pleasant, slightly sour aroma.
- **Warmth is Key:** Both sorghum and amaranth starters thrive in a consistently warm environment.

Using Your Starters in Bread

Once your sorghum or amaranth starter is bubbly and active, you have a few options:

- **Direct Use:** Use a portion of your mature starter directly in your gluten-free bread recipes.
- **Flavor Development:** Maintain and feed your starter regularly for continued flavor development before baking. The longer it matures, the more complex the taste will become.

Gluten-free sourdough starters can be slightly less predictable than traditional wheat-based ones. Be patient, experiment with flour blends, and soon you'll be mastering delicious loaves with these unique flours!

FAQs: All About Sourdough Starters

Q: How do I know if my sourdough starter is bad?

A: There are a few key signs that your starter might have spoiled:

- **Mold:** Any fuzzy spots (pink, green, orange, etc.) indicate mold growth. Unfortunately, mold has roots that extend below the surface, so if you see any, it's best to start fresh.
- **Unpleasant Odors:** A healthy starter can have a slightly sour, yeasty smell or even a touch of vinegar. However, a persistently foul, rotten smell could signal the presence of unwelcome bacteria.
- **Separation Without Revival:** If a layer of gray liquid (hooch) forms and normal feedings don't revive the starter with bubbly activity, it might be time to restart.

Q: Did I kill my sourdough starter?

A: Sourdough starters are remarkably resilient! Here are common worries and why you probably haven't killed your starter:

- **Forgot to Feed It:** Neglected starters might develop a thick layer of hooch and look sad, but they can often be revived. Pour off the hooch, discard some of the starter, and resume regular feedings. It should perk up!
- **Used the Wrong Flour:** A temporary change in flour won't destroy your starter. Resume your usual routine, and it'll adapt.
- **Temperature Fluctuations:** Oven warmth or a brief cold spell won't necessarily kill your starter. Be patient and observe it during regular feedings. Signs of life should return.

Q: My starter is bubbly but not rising. What's wrong?

A: Several factors might be at play:

- **Young Starter:** New starters need time to gain strength. Be patient and continue regular feedings.
- **Wet Mixture:** Try slightly reducing the water during feedings. A thicker consistency might encourage better rise.
- **Flour Choice:** Different flours offer varying levels of support. Experiment with blends for the right rise.
- **Cold Environment:** Starters thrive in warmth. Find a cozy spot for yourself and observe if the rise improves.

Q: Can I save a neglected refrigerated starter?

A: Absolutely! Even after a long refrigerator stint, your starter likely has viable yeast and bacteria. Follow these steps:

- **Inspect:** Discard any mold, as well as the gray, alcoholic liquid (hooch) on top. Look for a healthy, cream-colored starter layer below.
- **Revive:** Take a small portion (30g) and feed with equal parts flour and water. Keep it warm and observe. It might take a few feedings before regaining its bubbly enthusiasm.

Q: How do I make a backup of my starter?

A: Here's how to create a safety net through dehydration:

- **Spread:** Thinly spread a portion of your starter on parchment paper.
- **Dry:** Let it dry completely for a day or two in a draft-free area.
- **Store:** Break the dried starter into small pieces and store them in an airtight container in the pantry or freezer. Dehydrated starters can last for years!

Additional Tips:

- **Trust Your Senses:** Sourdough starters go through different smells as they develop. Learn to recognize the usual "yeasty" smell versus a truly off-putting one.
- **Document Your Journey:** Keep a notebook with feeding schedules, flour types, and observations. This helps you learn from both successes and minor setbacks.
- **Resources:** Explore online videos and blog posts for troubleshooting and inspiration. The sourdough community is amazingly helpful!

Chapter 4: The Zero-Waste Kitchen: Sourdough Discard Delights

Sweet Treats: Muffins (7 Recipes)

In the journey of sourdough baking, one often encounters the challenge of waste management—specifically, what to do with the leftover sourdough starter, commonly referred to as "discard." This chapter is dedicated to transforming what might otherwise be seen as waste into a treasure trove of culinary delights. Embracing a zero-waste approach not only aligns with sustainable cooking practices but also unlocks a myriad of delicious possibilities.

Sourdough discard, the portion of the starter that is removed before feeding, is still full of potential. Though it may lack the leavening power of a freshly fed starter, its tangy flavor is perfect for enhancing a variety of recipes. From breakfast to dinner and everything in between, sourdough discard can be incorporated into dishes that will surprise and delight any palate.

In this chapter, we explore recipes that utilize sourdough discard in creative and tasty ways. Whether you're making pancakes, waffles, crackers, or even cakes, these recipes will help you make the most of your sourdough starter. By integrating sourdough discard into your regular cooking routine, you contribute to a more sustainable kitchen practice, reducing waste and adding a unique flavor twist to everyday meals.

Prepare to discover how versatile your sourdough discard can be and how it can elevate the simplest recipes into something extraordinary. Each recipe in this chapter not only offers a chance to minimize kitchen waste but also enhances the nutritional value of your meals, making this approach a win-win for both your palate and the planet.

Let's dive into the world of sourdough discard and transform the way you think about your sourdough baking residues.

Recipe 1: Tropical Chia Powerhouse: Blend sourdough discard (sorghum or brown rice starter), mashed banana, passion fruit pulp, chia seeds, Greek yogurt, and a touch of honey.

Recipe 2: Sunrise Surprise Muffin: Combine sourdough discard (any variety), grated carrot, pumpkin seeds, unsweetened applesauce, spices (cinnamon, ginger), chopped apricots, and a scoop of protein powder.

Recipe 3: Almond Berry Burst: Mix sourdough discard (amaranth or millet starter complements the nutty flavor), mashed blueberries, almond flour, almond milk, egg, a hint of vanilla extract, and chopped almonds for crunch.

Recipe 4: Chocolate Avocado Delight: Blend sourdough discard, mashed avocado (provides healthy fats), unsweetened cocoa powder, egg, a small amount of maple syrup, and dark chocolate chips.

Recipe 5: Nutty Pear Spice: Combine sourdough discard, grated pear, chopped walnuts, egg, spices like cinnamon and nutmeg, and a touch of brown sugar.

Recipe 6: Savory Protein Kick: Sourdough discard, grated zucchini, chopped lean ham or cooked chicken, grated cheddar cheese, chives, and a dash of hot sauce. (Unexpected and savory, not sweet!)

Recipe 7: Raspberry & Quinoa Power: Mix sourdough discard, mashed raspberries, cooked quinoa, ground flaxseeds, egg, and a touch of honey or maple syrup.

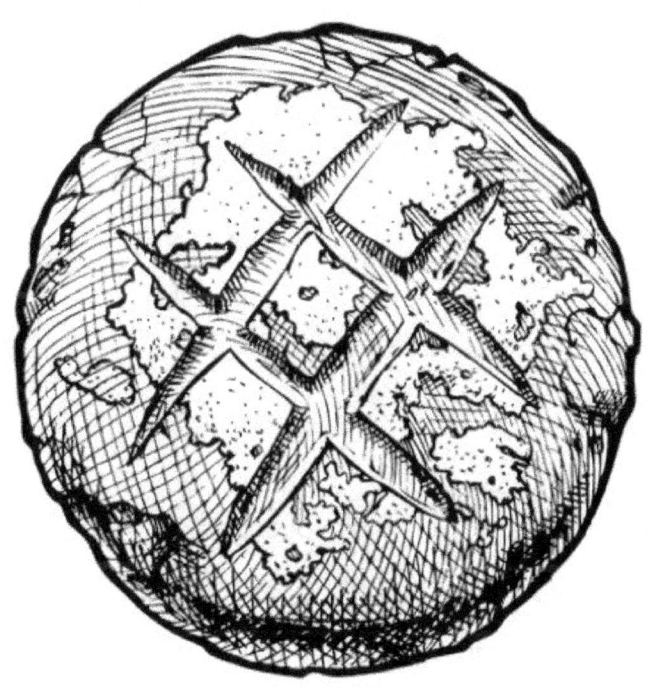

Recipe #1: Tropical Chia Powerhouse

Prep Time: 15 mins | **Cooking Time:** 18-22 mins | **Servings:** 12 muffins.

Why It's Essential: This muffin offers a delicious blend of tropical flavors, healthy fats from chia seeds, a protein boost from Greek yogurt, and the subtle tang of sourdough.

Ingredients:

- 1/2 cup sourdough discard (brown rice or sorghum starter for a neutral base)
- 1 ripe banana, mashed.
- 1/4 cup passion fruit pulp
- 2 tablespoons chia seeds
- 1/2 cup Greek yogurt (plain or vanilla)
- 1 tablespoon honey or maple syrup
- 1 large egg
- 1/2 cup gluten-free all-purpose flour
- 1/2 teaspoon baking soda
- 1/4 teaspoon baking powder
- 1/4 teaspoon salt

Optional Alternatives:

- Is passion fruit not available? Substitute mango or pineapple.
- For extra sweetness, add a sprinkle of shredded coconut.

Instructions:

1. **Preheat & Prep:** Preheat oven to 375°F (190°C). Line a muffin tin with paper liners or grease lightly.
2. **Mix Wet Ingredients:** Combine sourdough discard, banana, passion fruit, chia seeds, yogurt, honey, and egg.
3. **Whisk Dry Ingredients:** In a separate bowl, whisk together flour, baking soda, baking powder, and salt.
4. **Combine:** Add dry ingredients to the wet mixture, stirring until just combined (don't overmix).
5. **Bake:** Divide batter evenly among muffin cups. Bake for 18-22 minutes or until a toothpick inserted comes out clean.
6. **Cool:** Let muffins cool in the pan for a few minutes before transferring to a wire rack.

Nutritional Values (per serving):

- Calories: 150
- Carbohydrates: 20g
- Protein: 8g
- Fat: 6g
- Sodium: 120mg (approx.)
- Fiber: 3g

Cooking Tips:

- Use ripe bananas for optimal sweetness.
- Add a sprinkle of shredded coconut for an extra tropical touch.

Special Diets: This recipe can be adapted as follows:

- **Dairy-free:** Use a plant-based yogurt alternative.
- **Egg-free:** Substitute with a flax egg (1 tablespoon ground flaxseed + 3 tablespoons water).

Recipe #2: Sunrise Surprise Muffin

Prep Time: 15 mins | **Cooking Time:** 18-22 mins | **Servings:** 12 muffins.

Why It's Essential: This muffin is brimming with fiber, antioxidants, healthy fats, and a hint of sweetness. Perfect for a satisfying, energizing breakfast, or snack.

Ingredients:

- 1/2 cup sourdough discard (any variety works well)
- 1/2 cup grated carrot.
- 1/4 cup pumpkin seeds
- 1/4 cup unsweetened applesauce
- 1/4 teaspoon cinnamon
- 1/8 teaspoon ground ginger
- 1/4 cup chopped dried apricots.
- 1 scoop of protein powder (vanilla or unflavored)
- 1 large egg
- 1/4 cup gluten-free all-purpose flour
- 1/4 teaspoon baking soda
- 1/4 teaspoon baking powder
- Pinch of salt

Optional Alternatives:

- Swap pumpkin seeds for sunflower seeds or chopped walnuts.
- Use chopped dates or raisins instead of dried apricots.
- If you don't have protein powder, add an extra egg for protein.

Instructions:

5. **Preheat & Prep:** Preheat oven to 375°F (190°C). Line a muffin tin with paper liners or grease lightly.
6. **Combine Wet Ingredients:** In a bowl, mix sourdough discard, carrot, applesauce, spices, apricots, protein powder, and egg.
7. **Whisk Dry Ingredients:** In a separate bowl, whisk together flour, baking soda, baking powder, and salt.
8. **Combine:** Add dry ingredients to the wet mixture, stirring until just combined.
9. **Bake:** Divide batter evenly among the muffin cups. Bake for 18-22 minutes or until a toothpick inserted comes out clean.
10. **Cool:** Let muffins cool in the pan for a few minutes before transferring to a wire rack.

Nutritional Values:

- Calories: 160
- Carbohydrates: 22g
- Protein: 10g
- Fat: 5g
- Sodium: 100mg (approx.)
- Fiber: 4

Cooking Tips:

- Finely grate the carrots for even distribution within the muffin.
- For a touch of sweetness, drizzle a light honey glaze over the cooled muffins.

Special Diets:

- **Vegan:** Substitute the egg with a flax egg.

Recipe #3: Almond Berry Burst

Prep Time: 15 mins | **Cooking Time:** 18-22 mins | **Servings:** 12 muffins.

Why It's Essential: This muffin offers a delightful combination of almond and berry flavors with the subtle tang of sourdough. Perfect for a nourishing breakfast or snack.

Ingredients:

- 1/2 cup sourdough discard (amaranth or millet starter complements the nutty flavor)
- 1/2 cup mashed blueberries (or raspberries)
- 1/2 cup almond flour
- 1/4 cup almond milk
- 1 large egg
- 1 teaspoon vanilla extract
- 1/4 cup chopped almonds.
- 1/4 cup gluten-free all-purpose flour
- 1/4 teaspoon baking soda
- 1/4 teaspoon baking powder
- Pinch of salt

Optional Alternatives:

- Use your favorite berries - strawberries or blackberries work beautifully.
- Swap chopped almonds for pecans or walnuts.

Instructions:

1. **Preheat & Prep:** Preheat oven to 375°F (190°C). Line a muffin tin with paper liners or grease lightly.
2. **Combine Wet Ingredients:** In a bowl, mix sourdough, discard, mashed blueberries, almond flour, almond milk, egg, and vanilla extract.
3. **Whisk Dry Ingredients:** In a separate bowl, whisk together gluten-free flour, baking soda, baking powder, and salt.
4. **Combine:** Add dry ingredients to the wet mixture and stir until just combined. Fold in the chopped almonds.
5. **Bake:** Divide batter evenly among the muffin cups. Bake for 18-22 minutes or until a toothpick inserted comes out clean.
6. **Cool:** Let muffins cool in the pan for a few minutes before transferring to a wire rack.

Nutritional Values:

- ❖ Calories: 180
- ❖ Carbohydrates: 18g
- ❖ Protein: 7g
- ❖ Fat: 12g
- ❖ Sodium: 110mg (approx.)
- ❖ Fiber: 3g

Cooking Tips:

- ✓ Use fresh or frozen (thawed & drained) berries.
- ✓ Sprinkle a few slivered almonds on top before baking for added crunch.

Special Diets:

- **Dairy-free:** Use plant-based milk alternatives.

Recipe #4: Chocolate Avocado Delight

Prep Time: 15 mins | **Cooking Time:** 18-22 mins | **Servings:** 12 muffins!

Why It's Essential: This muffin delivers a decadent chocolate treat while incorporating healthy fats from avocado.

Ingredients:

- 1/2 cup sourdough discard (any variety)
- 1/2 ripe avocado, mashed.
- 1/4 cup unsweetened cocoa powder
- 1 large egg
- 1/4 cup maple syrup (or honey)
- 1/4 cup dark chocolate chips
- 1/4 cup gluten-free all-purpose flour
- 1/4 teaspoon baking soda
- 1/4 teaspoon baking powder
- Pinch of salt

Optional Alternatives:

- For a richer flavor, use melted coconut oil in place of maple syrup.
- Add a pinch of cinnamon or a dash of vanilla extract for extra depth.

Instructions:

1. Preheat & Prep: Preheat oven to 350°F (175°C). Line a muffin tin with paper liners or grease lightly.
2. Mix Wet Ingredients: Combine sourdough discard, avocado, cocoa powder, egg, maple syrup, and vanilla (if using).
3. Whisk Dry Ingredients: In a separate bowl, whisk together flour, baking soda, baking powder, and salt.
4. Combine: Add dry ingredients to the wet mixture and stir until just combined. Gently fold in the chocolate chips.
5. Bake: Divide batter evenly among the muffin cups. Bake for 18-22 minutes, or until a toothpick inserted comes out with a few moist crumbs.
6. Cool: Let muffins cool in the pan for a few minutes before transferring to a wire rack.

Nutritional Values:

- Calories: 170
- Carbohydrates: 20g
- Protein: 5g
- Fat: 10g
- Sodium: 90mg (approx.)
- Fiber: 4g

Cooking Tips:

- ✓ Ensure the avocado is very ripe for easy mashing.
- ✓ Use a higher percentage of cocoa in dark chocolate chips for a more intense chocolate flavor.

Special Diets:

- **Vegan**: Substitute the egg with a flax egg.

Recipe #5: Nutty Pear Spice

Prep Time: 15 mins | **Cooking Time:** 18-22 mins | **Servings:** 12 muffins.

Why It's Essential: This muffin offers cozy fall flavors with warm spices, the sweetness of pear, and a satisfying crunch from nuts.

Ingredients:

- 1/2 cup sourdough discard (any variety)
- 1/2 cup grated pear.
- 1/4 cup chopped walnuts.
- 1 large egg
- 1/4 teaspoon cinnamon
- 1/8 teaspoon ground nutmeg
- 1 tablespoon brown sugar
- 1/4 cup gluten-free all-purpose flour
- 1/4 teaspoon baking soda
- 1/4 teaspoon baking powder
- Pinch of salt

Optional Alternatives:

- Substitute walnuts with pecans or almonds.
- Add a touch of ground ginger or allspice for extra warmth.
- Swap brown sugar for a sprinkle of coconut sugar.

Instructions:

1. **Preheat & Prep:** Preheat oven to 375°F (190°C). Line a muffin tin with paper liners or grease lightly.
2. **Combine Wet Ingredients:** In a bowl, mix sourdough, discard, pear, walnuts, egg, spices, and brown sugar.
3. **Whisk Dry Ingredients:** In a separate bowl, whisk together flour, baking soda, baking powder, and salt.
4. **Combine:** Add dry ingredients to the wet mixture and stir until just combined.
5. **Bake:** Divide batter evenly among the muffin cups. Bake for 18-22 minutes or until a toothpick inserted comes out clean.
6. **Cool:** Let muffins cool in the pan for a few minutes before transferring to a wire rack.

Nutritional Values:

- Calories: 160
- Carbohydrates: 20g
- Protein: 6g
- Fat: 8g
- Sodium: 100mg (approx.)
- Fiber: 3g

Cooking Tips:

- Use a ripe pear for the best flavor and sweetness.
- For a streusel-like topping, mix a sprinkle of gluten-free flour, chopped walnuts, brown sugar, and a touch of cinnamon, then sprinkle it over the batter before baking.

Special Diets:

- **Vegan**: Substitute the egg with a flax egg.

Recipe #6: Savory Protein Kick

Prep Time: 15 mins | **Cook Time:** 18-22 mins | **Servings:** 12 muffins!

Why It's Essential: This savory muffin breaks the mold and provides a protein-packed, satisfying option for breakfast or snacks.

Ingredients:

- 1/2 cup sourdough discard (any variety)
- 1/2 cup grated zucchini.
- 1/4 cup chopped lean ham or cooked chicken.
- 1/4 cup grated cheddar cheese.
- 1 tablespoon chopped chives.
- Dash of hot sauce (optional)
- 1 large egg
- 1/4 cup gluten-free all-purpose flour
- 1/4 teaspoon baking powder
- 1/4 teaspoon baking soda
- Pinch of salt and black pepper

Optional Alternatives:

- Swap cheddar cheese for your favorite shredded cheese, like mozzarella or Swiss cheese.
- Add other chopped vegetables like bell peppers or mushrooms.
- Use crumbled cooked sausage instead of ham or chicken for a different flavor.

Instructions:

1. **Preheat & Prep:** Preheat oven to 375°F (190°C). Line a muffin tin with paper liners or grease lightly.
2. **Combine Wet Ingredients:** In a bowl, mix sourdough, discard, zucchini, ham or chicken, cheese, chives, hot sauce (if using), and egg.
3. **Whisk Dry Ingredients:** In a separate bowl, whisk together flour, baking powder, baking soda, salt, and pepper.
4. **Combine:** Add dry ingredients to the wet mixture and stir until just combined.
5. **Bake:** Divide batter evenly among the muffin cups. Bake for 18-22 minutes, or until a toothpick inserted comes out clean and the muffins are set.
6. **Cool:** Let muffins cool in the pan for a few minutes before transferring to a wire rack.

Nutritional Values:

- Calories: 180
- Carbohydrates: 15g
- Protein: 12g
- Fat: 10g
- Sodium: 350mg (approx.)
- Fiber: 2g

Cooking Tips:

- Squeeze excess moisture from the zucchini before adding it to the batter.
- Serve warm or at room temperature.
- These muffins are stored well in the refrigerator and can be reheated for a quick breakfast or snack.

Special Diets:

- **Vegetarian:** Substitute the ham or chicken with crumbled tofu or chopped mushrooms.

Recipe #7: Raspberry & Quinoa Power

Prep Time: 15 mins | **Cooking Time:** 18-22 mins | **Servings:** 12 muffins!

Why It's Essential: This muffin offers a boost of protein and antioxidants from the quinoa and raspberries, combined with the signature sourdough tang, for a unique and delicious breakfast or snack.

Ingredients:

- 1/2 cup sourdough discard (any variety)
- 1/2 cup mashed raspberries (fresh or frozen)
- 1/2 cup cooked quinoa
- 1/4 cup ground flaxseeds
- 1 large egg
- 1 tablespoon honey or maple syrup
- 1/4 cup gluten-free all-purpose flour
- 1/4 teaspoon baking soda
- 1/4 teaspoon baking powder
- Pinch of salt

Optional Alternatives:

- Use other berries like blueberries or blackberries.
- Add a sprinkle of cinnamon for a touch of warmth.

Instructions:

1. **Preheat & Prep:** Preheat oven to 375°F (190°C). Line a muffin tin with paper liners or grease lightly.
2. **Combine Wet Ingredients:** In a bowl, mix sourdough, discard, raspberries, quinoa, ground flaxseeds, egg, and honey or maple syrup.
3. **Whisk Dry Ingredients:** In a separate bowl, whisk together flour, baking soda, baking powder, and salt.
4. **Combine:** Add dry ingredients to the wet mixture and stir until just combined.
5. **Bake:** Divide batter evenly among the muffin cups. Bake for 18-22 minutes or until a toothpick inserted comes out clean.
6. **Cool:** Let muffins cool in the pan for a few minutes before transferring to a wire rack.

Nutritional Values:

- Calories: 150
- Carbohydrates: 22g
- Protein: 8g
- Fat: 5g
- Sodium: 90mg (approx.)
- Fiber: 4g

Cooking Tips:

- ✓ If using frozen raspberries, thaw and drain them before adding to the batter.
- ✓ Serve with a dollop of Greek yogurt for an added protein boost.

Special Diets:

- **Vegan:** Substitute the egg with a flax egg.

Chapter 5: Pancakes & Waffles (6 Recipes)

Introduction to Chapter 5: Pancakes & Waffles

Breakfast is often called the most important meal of the day, and what better way to elevate your morning routine than by incorporating the unique flavors and textures of sourdough into classic breakfast staples? Chapter 5 is dedicated to transforming your breakfast table with a delightful assortment of sourdough pancakes and waffles. Each recipe harnesses the tangy complexity of sourdough to add a new dimension to these beloved dishes.

This chapter will guide you through six inventive recipes that range from light and fluffy pancakes to crispy, golden waffles, each with a sourdough twist. Whether you're looking for a simple, comforting meal to start your day or something special for a weekend brunch, these recipes provide versatile options that cater to various tastes and preferences.

We'll explore different techniques to incorporate sourdough starter into pancake and waffle batters, ensuring you achieve the perfect texture and flavor. Additionally, tips on how to customize your pancakes and waffles with a variety of mix-ins and toppings will be provided, allowing you to personalize each dish to your liking.

Prepare to delight your family and friends with recipes that not only taste incredible but also add a nutritional boost from the natural fermentation of sourdough. From hearty, whole-grain options to decadently sweet treats, these pancakes and waffles are sure to become a cherished part of your culinary repertoire.

Let's dive into the world of sourdough breakfasts and start your day with a smile!

Recipe 8: Protein-Packed Pumpkin Power: Combine sourdough discard (sorghum or brown rice starter), pumpkin puree, protein powder, eggs, spices (cinnamon, nutmeg), and a touch of maple syrup.

Recipe 9: Fluffy Banana & Greek Yogurt: Blend sourdough discard, mashed banana, Greek yogurt, egg, a dash of vanilla, and a sprinkle of oats for texture.

Recipe 10: Kiwi Chia Burst: Mix sourdough discard, mashed kiwi fruit, chia seeds, egg, almond milk, and a hint of honey or maple syrup.

Recipe 11: Jackfruit & Coconut Surprise: Combine sourdough discard (millet or amaranth starter), mashed jackfruit (unique texture), shredded coconut, egg, coconut milk, and a touch of brown sugar.

Recipe 12: Carrot Cake Fusion: Blend sourdough discard, grated carrot, walnuts, spices (cinnamon, ginger), egg, applesauce, and a touch of molasses for depth.

Recipe 13: Savory Ricotta & Herb: Combine sourdough discard, ricotta cheese, chopped herbs (basil, parsley, chives), grated parmesan, egg, and a pinch of salt & pepper.

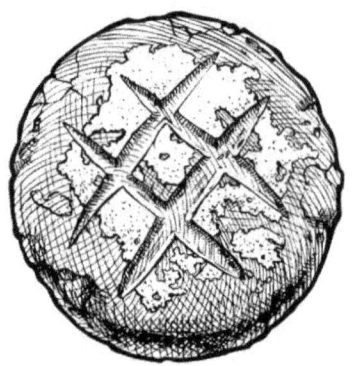

***Temperature Matters**: "Maintain a warm environment, ideally between 75°F and 80°F, during the fermentation process to encourage active yeast and bacterial growth in your sourdough."*

Recipe 8: Protein-Packed Pumpkin Power

Prep Time: 10 mins | **Cook Time:** 3-4 mins per pancake/waffle | **Servings:** 4-6

Why It's Essential: This recipe offers a protein-fueled, fiber-rich, and flavor-packed twist on classic pancakes or waffles. Perfect for a post-workout breakfast or a satisfying weekend brunch.

Ingredients:

- 1 cup sourdough discard (brown rice or sorghum starter for a neutral base)
- 1/2 cup pumpkin puree
- 1 scoop protein powder (vanilla or unflavored)
- 2 large eggs
- 1 teaspoon cinnamon
- 1/2 teaspoon nutmeg
- 1/4 teaspoon ginger powder (optional)
- 1 tablespoon maple syrup
- 1/4 teaspoon baking soda
- Pinch of salt

Step-by-Step Instructions:

1. **Whisk Wet Ingredients:** Combine sourdough discard, pumpkin puree, protein powder, eggs, spices, maple syrup, baking soda, and salt. Whisk until smooth.
2. **Cook:** Lightly grease a skillet or waffle iron and heat over medium heat.
3. **For pancakes:** Pour 1/4 cup batter per pancake onto the hot skillet. Cook until bubbles form on the surface and the edges look set, then flip and cook the other side until golden brown.
4. **For waffles:** Follow the instructions for your specific waffle iron.
5. **Serve:** Serve warm with your favorite toppings like maple syrup, fresh berries, whipped cream, nuts, or a drizzle of nut butter.

Nutritional Values (per serving):

- ❖ Calories: 200
- ❖ Carbohydrates: 25g
- ❖ Protein: 20g
- ❖ Fat: 7g
- ❖ Sodium: 250mg
- ❖ Fiber: 4g

Cooking Tips:

- ✓ Use ripe pumpkin puree for the best flavor and sweetness.
- ✓ Adjust the spice mix to your liking.
- ✓ If the batter is too thick, add a splash of milk (dairy or plant-based).

Special Diets:

- **Vegan:** Substitute the eggs with 2 flax eggs (2 tablespoons ground flaxseed + 6 tablespoons water).
- **Dairy-free:** Use plant-based milk if needed to adjust the batter consistency.

Recipe 9: Fluffy Banana & Greek Yogurt

Prep Time: 10 mins | **Cook Time:** 3-4 mins per pancake/waffle | **Servings:** 4-6

Why It's Essential: This recipe boasts a delightful combination of banana, Greek yogurt, and the subtle tang of sourdough. It delivers a fluffy texture that is perfect for a cozy breakfast.

Ingredients:

- 1 cup sourdough discard (any variety works well)
- 1 ripe banana, mashed.
- 1/2 cup Greek yogurt (plain or vanilla)
- 1 large egg
- 1 teaspoon vanilla extract
- 1/4 cup rolled oats.
- 1/4 cup gluten-free all-purpose flour
- 1/4 teaspoon baking soda
- 1/4 teaspoon baking powder
- Pinch of salt

Step-by-Step Instructions:

1. **Blend Wet Ingredients:** In a blender or bowl, combine sourdough discard, mashed banana, Greek yogurt, egg, and vanilla extract. Blend or whisk until smooth.
2. **Add Dry Ingredients:** Add rolled oats, flour, baking soda, baking powder, and salt to the wet ingredients. Mix gently until just combined.
3. **Cook:** Lightly grease a skillet or waffle iron and heat over medium heat. Follow the same cooking instructions as in Recipe #1 for either pancakes or waffles.
4. **Serve:** Serve warm with your choice of toppings (e.g., fresh fruit, maple syrup, a dollop of yogurt, nuts).

Nutritional Values (per serving):

- ❖ Calories: 180
- ❖ Carbohydrates: 28g
- ❖ Protein: 10g
- ❖ Fat: 6g
- ❖ Sodium: 200mg
- ❖ Fiber: 4g

Cooking Tips:

- ✓ Use a very ripe banana for optimal sweetness and easy blending.
- ✓ For extra thickness, let the batter rest for 5 minutes before cooking.

Special Diets:

- **Vegan:** Substitute the egg with a flax egg (1 tablespoon ground flaxseed + 3 tablespoons water).
- **Dairy-free:** Use plant-based yogurt.

Recipe 10: Kiwi Chia Burst

Prep Time: 10 mins | **Cook Time:** 3-4 mins per pancake/waffle | **Servings:** 4-6

Why It's Essential: This recipe offers a refreshing tropical twist with kiwi, a boost of healthy fats from chia seeds, and the unique flavor of sourdough for a tasty and nutritious option.

Ingredients:

- 1 cup sourdough discard (any variety)
- 2 ripe kiwis peeled and mashed.
- 1/4 cup chia seeds
- 1 large egg
- 1/4 cup almond milk (or milk of choice)
- 1 tablespoon honey or maple syrup
- 1/4 cup gluten-free all-purpose flour
- 1/4 teaspoon baking soda
- 1/4 teaspoon baking powder
- Pinch of salt

Step-by-Step Instructions:

1. **Combine Wet Ingredients:** In a bowl, whisk together sourdough discard, mashed kiwi, chia seeds, egg, almond milk, and sweetener of choice. Let sit for a few minutes to allow the chia seeds to soften.
2. **Add Dry Ingredients:** Add flour, baking soda, baking powder, and salt to the wet ingredients. Stir gently until just combined.
3. **Cook:** Lightly grease a skillet or waffle iron and heat over medium heat. Follow the same instructions as in Recipe #1 for either pancakes or waffles.
4. **Serve:** Serve warm with your favorite toppings like fresh kiwi slices, berries, a drizzle of honey, or a sprinkle of shredded coconut.

Nutritional Values (per serving):

- Calories: 160
- Carbohydrates: 24g
- Protein: 7g
- Fat: 7g
- Sodium: 180mg
- Fiber: 5g

Cooking Tips:

- If you don't have fresh kiwi, frozen kiwi (thawed and well-drained) can work in a pinch.
- Add a sprinkle of cinnamon for a touch of warmth.

Special Diets:

- **Vegan:** Substitute the egg with a flax egg (1 tablespoon ground flaxseed + 3 tablespoons water).
- **Dairy-free:** Ensure you use a plant-based milk alternative.

Recipe 11: Jackfruit & Coconut Surprise

Prep Time: 15 mins | **Cook Time:** 3-4 mins per pancake/waffle | **Servings:** 4-6

Why It's Essential: This recipe offers a unique and flavorful experience with the interesting texture of jackfruit, sweetness from coconut, and the subtle tang of sourdough.

Ingredients:

- 1 cup sourdough discard (millet or amaranth starter complements the tropical flavors)
- 1/2 cup mashed jackfruit (canned in water or brine, drained and rinsed)
- 1/4 cup shredded coconut
- 1 large egg
- 1/4 cup coconut milk (or milk of choice)
- 1 tablespoon brown sugar
- 1/4 cup gluten-free all-purpose flour
- 1/4 teaspoon baking soda
- 1/4 teaspoon baking powder
- Pinch of salt

Alternative Ingredients:

- Is Jackfruit not available? Substitute mashed mango or pineapple for a similar tropical sweetness.

Step-by-Step Instructions:

1. **Combine Wet Ingredients:** In a bowl, whisk together sourdough discard, mashed jackfruit, shredded coconut, egg, coconut milk, and brown sugar.
2. **Add Dry Ingredients:** Add flour, baking soda, baking powder, and salt to the wet ingredients. Stir gently until just combined.
3. **Cook:** Lightly grease a skillet or waffle iron and heat over medium heat. Follow the same instructions as in Recipe #1 for either pancakes or waffles.
4. **Serve:** Serve warm with your favorite toppings like toasted coconut flakes, fresh fruit, a drizzle of honey, or a dollop of whipped cream.

Nutritional Values (per serving):

- ❖ Calories: 190
- ❖ Carbohydrates: 28g
- ❖ Protein: 6g
- ❖ Fat: 8g
- ❖ Sodium: 190mg
- ❖ Fiber: 3g

Cooking Tips:

- ✓ Make sure to use unsweetened shredded coconut for the best flavor balance.
- ✓ If the batter seems too thin, add a little more gluten-free flour.

Special Diets:

- **Vegan**: Substitute the egg with a flax egg (1 tablespoon ground flaxseed + 3 tablespoons water).
- **Dairy-free**: Ensure you use a plant-based milk alternative.

Recipe 12: Carrot Cake Fusion

Prep Time: 15 mins | **Cook Time:** 3-4 mins per pancake/waffle | **Servings:** 4-6

Why It's Essential: This recipe brings the beloved flavors of carrot cake into a satisfying breakfast or snack, with added nutrition from walnuts, warming spices, and the signature sourdough tang.

Ingredients:

- 1 cup sourdough discard (any variety)
- 1/2 cup grated carrot.
- 1/4 cup chopped walnuts.
- 1 large egg
- 1/4 cup applesauce (unsweetened)
- 1 teaspoon cinnamon
- 1/2 teaspoon ginger powder
- 1 tablespoon molasses (or maple syrup)
- 1/4 cup gluten-free all-purpose flour
- 1/4 teaspoon baking soda
- 1/4 teaspoon baking powder
- Pinch of salt

Alternative Ingredients:

- Swap walnuts or, pecans or almonds.

Step-by-Step Instructions:

1. **Combine Wet Ingredients:** In a bowl, whisk together sourdough discard, grated carrot, walnuts, egg, applesauce, spices, and molasses (or maple syrup).
2. **Add Dry Ingredients:** Add flour, baking soda, baking powder, and salt to the wet ingredients. Stir gently until just combined.
3. **Cook:** Lightly grease a skillet or waffle iron and heat over medium heat. Follow the same instructions as in Recipe #1 for either pancakes or waffles.
4. **Serve:** Serve warm with your favorite toppings like cream cheese frosting (regular or dairy-free), chopped nuts, a sprinkle of cinnamon, or a dollop of yogurt.

Nutritional Values (per serving):

- Calories: 200
- Carbohydrates: 25g
- Protein: 8g
- Fat: 10g
- Sodium: 180mg
- Fiber: 4g

Cooking Tips:

- Finely grate the carrots to evenly distribute them in the batter.
- For a hint of sweetness, add a drizzle of maple syrup or honey over the cooked pancakes or waffles.

Special Diets:

- **Vegan**: Substitute the egg with a flax egg (1 tablespoon ground flaxseed + 3 tablespoons water).
- **Nut-free**: Omit the walnuts or substitute with sunflower seeds or pumpkin seeds.

Recipe 13: Savory Ricotta & Herb

Prep Time: 15 mins | **Cook Time:** 3-4 mins per pancake/waffle | **Servings:** 4-6

Why It's Essential: This recipe offers a unique and satisfying savory breakfast or brunch option, packed with the creamy richness of ricotta, fresh herbs, and a hint of tang from sourdough.

Ingredients:

- 1 cup sourdough discard (any variety)
- 1/2 cup ricotta cheese
- 1/4 cup chopped fresh herbs (basil, parsley, chives, or a combination)
- 1/4 cup grated parmesan cheese.
- 1 large egg
- 1/4 cup gluten-free all-purpose flour
- 1/4 teaspoon baking powder
- 1/4 teaspoon baking soda
- Pinch of salt and black pepper

Alternative Ingredients:

- Substitute ricotta for cottage cheese or thick Greek yogurt for a similar texture.
- Use your favorite combination of fresh herbs.

Step-by-Step Instructions:

1. **Combine Wet Ingredients:** In a bowl, whisk together sourdough discard, ricotta cheese, herbs, parmesan cheese, egg, and a pinch of salt and pepper.
2. **Add Dry Ingredients:** Add flour, baking powder, and baking soda to the wet ingredients. Stir gently until just combined.
3. **Cook:** Lightly grease a skillet or waffle iron and heat over medium heat. Follow the same instructions as in Recipe #1 for either pancakes or waffles.
4. **Serve:** Serve warm with your favorite savory toppings like a fried or poached egg, smoked salmon, chopped tomatoes, avocado, a sprinkle of red pepper flakes, or a dollop of pesto.

Nutritional Values (per serving):

- ❖ Calories: 220
- ❖ Carbohydrates: 18g
- ❖ Protein: 15g
- ❖ Fat: 10g
- ❖ Sodium: 400mg
- ❖ Fiber: 2g

Cooking Tips:

- ✓ If the batter seems too thick, add a splash of milk or water to thin it slightly.
- ✓ Top with a squeeze of lemon juice to brighten the flavor.

Special Diets:

- **Vegetarian**: This recipe is already vegetarian-friendly!

Chapter 6: Bread Pudding (4 Recipes)

Chapter 6 delves into the comforting world of bread pudding, transforming day-old sourdough bread into warm, custardy delights. This chapter features four unique recipes that showcase the versatility and richness of bread pudding, each using sourdough as a key ingredient to enhance the texture and flavor of this classic dessert.

Bread pudding, with its humble beginnings as a frugal way to use up stale bread, has evolved into a beloved comfort food enjoyed in various forms around the world. In this chapter, we breathe new life into sourdough scraps by soaking them in rich, flavorful custards infused with everything from classic vanilla and cinnamon to inventive mix-ins like chocolate, fruits, and nuts.

Each recipe in this chapter is designed to be approachable, whether you're a seasoned baker or new to the art of dessert making. You'll learn how to create moist, flavorful bread puddings that can serve as the centerpiece of a festive brunch or a cozy family dinner. Moreover, these recipes are adaptable, offering suggestions for substitutions and additions that allow you to customize the dishes according to your taste preferences and what you have on hand in your kitchen.

From a decadent chocolate espresso bread pudding to a bright, citrus-infused version, each dish promises to deliver comfort and satisfaction. We'll also include tips on achieving the perfect texture—neither too soggy nor too dry—and ideas for complementary sauces and toppings to make your bread puddings truly exceptional.

Prepare to indulge in the simple pleasures of baking as we explore the transformative magic that occurs when sourdough bread meets sweet, creamy custard.

Let's get ready to turn leftover bread into luscious treats that warm the heart and delight the palate.

Recipe 14: Spiced Pear Delight: Cube slightly stale gluten-free bread, toss with chopped pear spices, drizzle a mix of sourdough discard, egg, almond milk, and a touch of maple syrup. Bake until golden.

Recipe 15: Tropical Twist: Use cubed gluten-free bread, mix with diced mango, passion fruit pulp, coconut flakes, and custard of sourdough discard, coconut milk, eggs, and a hint of sweetener.

Recipe 16: Berry Burst: Cube bread, mix with blueberries and raspberries. Create a custard with sourdough discard, eggs, Greek yogurt, a dash of vanilla, and honey.

Recipe 17: Chocolate & Cherry Indulgence: Use cubed bread, toss with pitted cherries, chocolate chips, and a decadent custard of sourdough discard, eggs, unsweetened cocoa, and a touch of sugar.

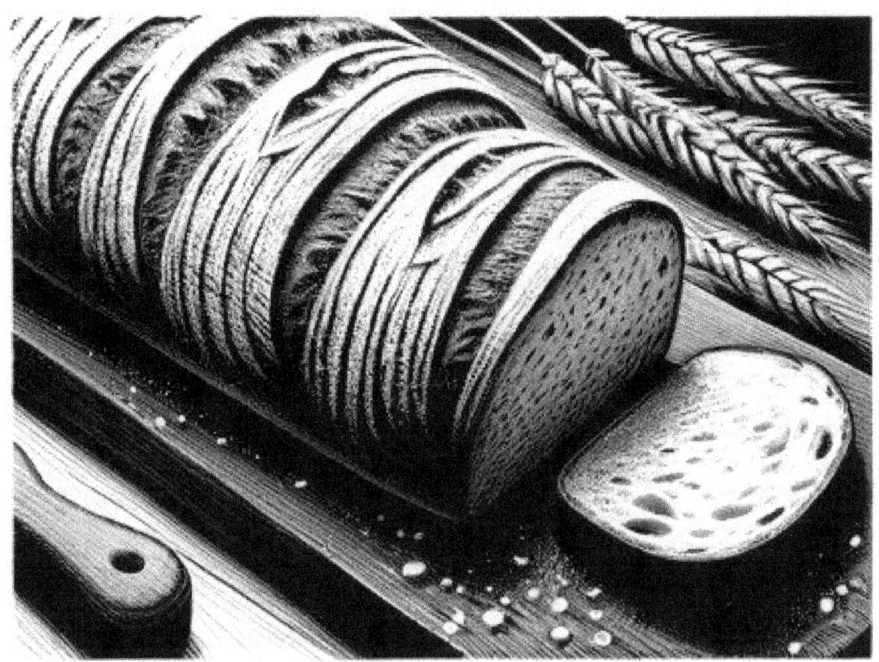

Autolyse for Better Texture: "Allow your mixed dough to rest for at least 30 minutes before adding salt and starter. This autolyse process helps develop gluten, leading to better texture and volume in your bread."

Recipe 14: Spiced Pear Delight

Prep Time: 15 mins | **Cook Time:** 30-35 mins | **Servings:** 6-8

Why It's Essential: This recipe offers a cozy autumnal feel with warm spices, the sweetness of pears, and the classic comfort of bread pudding, enhanced by the tang of sourdough.

Ingredients:

- 4 cups cubed, slightly stale gluten-free bread.
- 1 large ripe pear, diced.
- 1 teaspoon cinnamon
- 1/2 teaspoon ground nutmeg
- 1/4 teaspoon ground ginger (optional)
- 1/2 cup sourdough discard (any variety)
- 2 large eggs
- 1 cup almond milk (or milk of choice)
- 1/4 cup maple syrup
- 1 teaspoon vanilla extract

Step-by-Step Instructions:

1. **Prep:** Preheat oven to 350°F (175°C). Grease a 9x13-inch baking dish.
2. **Combine Bread & Fruit:** In a large bowl, toss together cubed bread, diced pear, and spices.
3. **Make Custard:** Whisk together sourdough discard, eggs, almond milk, maple syrup, and vanilla extract.
4. **Assemble:** Pour the custard mixture over the bread and pear mixture, making sure the bread is evenly coated. Let it soak for a few minutes.
5. **Bake:** Bake for 30-35 minutes, or until the custard is set and the top is golden brown.
6. **Serve:** Serve warm with a dollop of whipped cream, Greek yogurt, or a drizzle of maple syrup.

Nutritional Values (per serving):

- Calories: 250
- Carbohydrates: 38g
- Protein: 8g
- Fat: 10g
- Sodium: 150mg
- Fiber: 4g

Cooking Tips:

- Use slightly stale bread; it will soak up the custard more effectively.
- For extra sweetness, add a sprinkle of brown sugar over the top before baking.

Special Diets:

- **Vegan**: Use a plant-based milk alternative and substitute eggs with flax eggs (2 tablespoons ground flaxseed + 6 tablespoons water).
- **Dairy-free**: Ensure you use dairy-free milk.

Recipe 15: Tropical Twist

Prep Time: 15 mins | **Cook Time:** 30-35 mins | **Servings:** 6-8

Why It's Essential: This recipe brings vibrant tropical flavors of mango, passion fruit, and coconut together in a decadent bread pudding, perfect for a summery treat or a touch of sunshine any time of year.

Ingredients:

- 4 cups cubed, slightly stale gluten-free bread.
- 1 cup diced mango.
- 1/4 cup passion fruit pulp
- 1/4 cup shredded coconut
- 1/2 cup sourdough discard (any variety)
- 2 large eggs
- 1 cup coconut milk
- 1 tablespoon honey or maple syrup
- 1 teaspoon vanilla extract

Step-by-Step Instructions:

1. **Prep**: Preheat oven to 350°F (175°C). Grease a 9x13-inch baking dish.
2. **Combine Bread & Fruit:** In a large bowl, toss together cubed bread, diced mango, passion fruit pulp, and shredded coconut.
3. **Make Custard:** Whisk together sourdough discard, eggs, coconut milk, honey or maple syrup, and vanilla extract.
4. **Assemble:** Pour the custard mixture over the bread and fruit mixture. Ensure the bread is evenly coated, and let it soak for a few minutes.
5. **Bake**: Bake for 30-35 minutes, or until the custard is set and the top is golden brown.
6. **Serve**: Serve warm or at room temperature. Top with toasted coconut flakes or a drizzle of honey for an extra touch.

Nutritional Values (per serving):

- Calories: 280
- Carbohydrates: 35g
- Protein: 7g
- Fat: 15g
- Sodium: 120mg
- Fiber: 3g

Cooking Tips:

- Use fresh or frozen mango, thawed and drained.
- If you can't find passion fruit pulp, substitute it with a blend of pineapple juice and lime juice.

Special Diets:

- **Vegan**: Use a plant-based milk alternative and substitute eggs with flax eggs (2 tablespoons ground flaxseed + 6 tablespoons water).

Recipe 16: Berry Burst

Prep Time: 15 mins | **Cook Time:** 30-35 mins | **Servings:** 6-8

Why It's Essential: This recipe offers a naturally sweet and refreshing treat packed with antioxidants from berries and a protein boost from Greek yogurt in the custard.

Ingredients:

- 4 cups cubed slightly stale gluten-free bread (preferably made with your sorghum or brown rice sourdough starter)
- 1 cup mixed berries (blueberries, raspberries, or a combination)
- 1/2 cup sourdough discard (brown rice or sorghum starter is ideal)
- 2 large eggs
- 1 cup Greek yogurt (nonfat or low-fat)
- 1/4 cup honey or maple syrup
- 1 teaspoon vanilla extract

Alternative Ingredients

- If fresh berries aren't in season, use frozen berries, thawed and drained.
- Substitute Greek yogurt with a thick, unsweetened plant-based yogurt for a dairy-free option.

Step-by-Step Instructions:

1. **Prep:** Preheat oven to 350°F (175°C). Grease a 9x13-inch baking dish.
2. **Combine Bread & Fruit:** In a large bowl, toss together cubed bread and berries.
3. **Make Custard:** Whisk together sourdough discard, eggs, Greek yogurt, honey or maple syrup, and vanilla extract.
4. **Assemble:** Pour the custard mixture over the bread and berry mixture, ensuring the bread is evenly coated. Let it soak for a few minutes.
5. **Bake:** Bake for 30-35 minutes, or until the custard is set and the top is golden brown.
6. **Serve:** Serve warm or at room temperature. Top with a dollop of Greek yogurt and a sprinkle of fresh berries for an extra touch.

Nutritional Values (per serving):

- ❖ Calories: 220
- ❖ Carbohydrates: 30g
- ❖ Protein: 12g
- ❖ Fat: 7g
- ❖ Sodium: 100mg
- ❖ Fiber: 4g

Cooking Tips:

- ✓ Use a mix of berries for a vibrant flavor profile.
- ✓ Don't overbake! The custard should be set but still slightly jiggly in the center.

Special Diets:

- **Vegan**: Use a plant-based yogurt alternative and substitute eggs with flax eggs (2 tablespoons ground flaxseed + 6 tablespoons water).

Recipe 17: Chocolate & Cherry Indulgence

Prep Time: 15 mins | **Cook Time:** 30-35 mins | **Servings:** 6-8

Why It's Essential: This recipe offers a rich and satisfying flavor combination of chocolate and cherries, with the unique tang of sourdough adding depth. Perfect for a special treat or dessert.

Ingredients:

- 4 cups cubed, slightly stale gluten-free bread.
- 1/2 cup pitted cherries (fresh or frozen)
- 1/4 cup dark chocolate chips
- 1/2 cup sourdough discard (any variety works well)
- 2 large eggs
- 1/4 cup unsweetened cocoa powder
- 1/4 cup milk (dairy or plant-based)
- 1/4 cup sugar (or alternative sweetener)
- 1 teaspoon vanilla extract

Alternative Ingredients:

- Swap cherries with other tart fruits like cranberries or raspberries.

Step-by-Step Instructions:

1. **Prep:** Preheat oven to 350°F (175°C). Grease a 9x13-inch baking dish.
2. **Combine Bread, Fruit, & Chocolate:** In a large bowl, toss together cubed bread, cherries, and chocolate chips.
3. **Make Custard:** Whisk together sourdough discard, eggs, cocoa powder, milk, sugar, and **vanilla** extract.
4. Assemble: Pour the custard mixture over the bread mixture, ensuring the bread is evenly coated. Let it soak for a few minutes.
5. **Bake:** Bake for 30-35 minutes, or until the custard is set and the top is slightly puffed.
6. **Serve:** Serve warm with a scoop of vanilla ice cream (dairy or non-dairy), a drizzle of chocolate sauce, or a dusting of cocoa powder.

Nutritional Values (per serving):

- Calories: 280
- Carbohydrates: 40g
- Protein: 8g
- Fat: 12g
- Sodium: 130mg
- Fiber: 3g

Cooking Tips:

- Use a higher percentage of cocoa powder in your chocolate chips for a more intense chocolate flavor.
- Let the bread soak in the custard for a few minutes for optimal absorption.

Special Diets:

- **Vegan**: Use a plant-based milk alternative, substitute eggs with flax eggs (2 tablespoons ground flaxseed + 6 tablespoons water) and ensure your chocolate chips are dairy-free.

Chapter 7: Cookies (8 Recipes)

Welcome to a sweet chapter dedicated to one of everyone's favorite treats—cookies! Here, we explore eight unique cookie recipes, each with a twist that sets them apart from your everyday cookie jar staples. This chapter is all about versatility and creativity, utilizing various flavors, textures, and ingredients to elevate the humble cookie into a delightful gourmet experience.

Cookies are the perfect canvas for bakers to experiment with, and in this chapter, we do just that. From chewy to crispy, chocolatey to fruity, each recipe is designed to offer something special. Whether you're looking for a comforting classic with a new spin or something entirely innovative, these recipes are sure to inspire and excite.

We'll guide you through each step, from selecting the right ingredients to mixing and baking techniques that ensure perfect results every time. Each recipe also offers tips for customization, allowing you to adapt them to suit dietary preferences or to work with what you have available in your pantry.

In addition to traditional favorites, expect to find recipes that incorporate unexpected ingredients that harmonize beautifully with the basic components of cookies. We'll explore how to infuse flavors through spices, nuts, and extracts and how different textures can be achieved through the manipulation of ingredients and baking times.

Get ready to preheat your oven and prepare for the irresistible aroma of freshly baked cookies to fill your home. This chapter is not just about following recipes; it's about sparking creativity in the kitchen, sharing delicious results with loved ones, and enjoying the process of baking as much as the cookies themselves.

Let's dive into the dough and begin our cookie adventure!

Recipe 18: Oatmeal Apricot Power: Combine sourdough discard, oats, mashed dried apricots, ground flaxseeds, egg, and a touch of maple syrup.

Recipe 19: Nutty Chocolate Chip: Mix sourdough discard, almond flour, cashew butter, chocolate chips, egg, and a hint of vanilla.

Recipe 20: Pumpkin Seed & Spice: Combine sourdough discard, pumpkin puree, pumpkin seeds, ground flaxseed, spices, and a touch of molasses.

Recipe 21: Banana Chia Bites: Mash bananas, sourdough discard, chia seeds, oats, a touch of honey, and a sprinkle of cinnamon.

Recipe 22: PB & J Swirl: Mix sourdough discard, peanut butter, mashed raspberries, almond flour, egg, and a drizzle of honey.

Recipe 23: Blueberry Lemon Zest: Combine sourdough discard, almond flour, mashed blueberries, lemon zest, egg, and a hint of honey.

Recipe 24: Tropical Coconut Bites: Mix sourdough discard, shredded coconut, finely diced pineapple, ground macadamia nuts, and a touch of sweetener.

Recipe 25: Double Chocolate Delight: Combine sourdough discard, unsweetened cocoa, almond flour, chocolate chips, egg, and a touch of maple syrup.

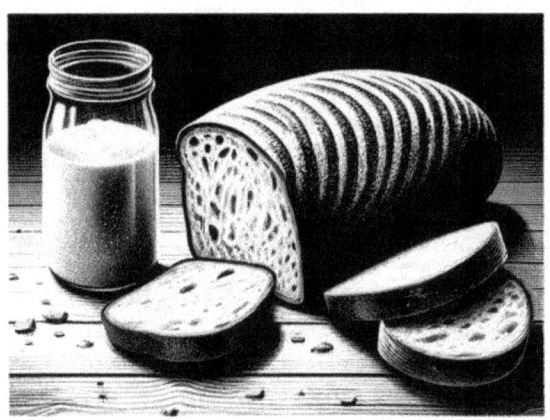

***Stretch and Fold for Strength**: "Perform several stretch and fold techniques during the first few hours of bulk fermentation to build strength in the dough without over-kneading."*

Recipe 18: Oatmeal Apricot Power

Prep Time: 10 mins | **Cook Time:** 12-15 mins per batch | **Servings:** 12-15 cookies

Ingredients:

- 1/2 cup sourdough discard (brown rice or sorghum starter is ideal)
- 1/2 cup rolled oats.
- 1/4 cup mashed dried apricots (or chopped dates)
- 1/4 cup ground flaxseeds
- 1 large egg
- 2 tablespoons maple syrup
- 1/4 teaspoon cinnamon
- Pinch of salt

Alternative Ingredients:

- Swap dried apricots for other dried fruits like raisins or cranberries.

Step-by-Step Instructions:

1. **Combine Ingredients:** In a bowl, mix sourdough discard, oats, mashed apricots, flaxseeds, egg, maple syrup, cinnamon, and salt.
2. **Chill (Optional): For** thicker cookies, chill the dough for 30 minutes.
3. **Shape & Bake:** Preheat oven to 350°F (175°C). Drop rounded tablespoons of dough onto a baking sheet lined with parchment paper. Bake for 12-15 minutes or until golden brown around the edges.
4. **Cool:** Let cookies cool on the baking sheet for a few minutes before transferring to a wire rack to cool completely.

Nutritional Values (per cookie):

- Calories: 90
- Carbohydrates: 12g
- Protein: 4g
- Fat: 4g
- Sodium: 30mg
- Fiber: 2

Cooking Tips:

- Soak dried apricots in hot water for a few minutes for easy mashing.
- For softer cookies, bake for a slightly shorter time.

Special Diets:

- **Vegan**: Substitute the egg with a flax egg (1 tablespoon ground flaxseed + 3 tablespoons water).

Recipe 19: Nutty Chocolate Chip

Prep Time: 10 mins | **Cook Time:** 12-15 mins per batch | **Servings:** 12-15 cookies!

Ingredients:

- 1/2 cup sourdough discard (any variety works well)
- 1/2 cup almond flour
- 1/4 cup cashew butter (or other nut butter)
- 1/4 cup chocolate chips (dark or semi-sweet)
- 1 large egg
- 1 teaspoon vanilla extract
- 1/4 teaspoon baking soda
- Pinch of salt

Alternative Ingredients:

- Swap cashew butter for peanut butter, sunflower seed butter, or another nut butter of choice.

Step-by-Step Instructions:

1. **Combine Ingredients:** In a bowl, mix sourdough discard, almond flour, cashew butter, chocolate chips, egg, vanilla extract, baking soda, and salt.
2. **Chill (Optional):** For thicker cookies, chill the dough for 30 minutes.
3. **Shape & Bake:** Preheat oven to 350°F (175°C). Drop rounded tablespoons of dough onto a baking sheet lined with parchment paper. Bake for 12-15 minutes or until golden brown around the edges.
4. **Cool:** Let cookies cool on the baking sheet for a few minutes before transferring to a wire rack to cool completely.

Nutritional Values (per cookie):

- Calories: 120
- Carbohydrates: 9g
- Protein: 5g
- Fat: 8g
- Sodium: 50mg
- Fiber: 2g

Cooking Tips:

- Use good quality cashew butter for optimal flavor.
- For a crunchier texture, add a sprinkle of chopped nuts to the dough.

Special Diets:

- **Vegan**: Substitute the egg with a flax egg (1 tablespoon ground flaxseed + 3 tablespoons water). Ensure chocolate chips are dairy-free.
- **Gluten-free:** This recipe is already gluten-free!

Recipe 20: Pumpkin Seed & Spice

Prep Time: 10 mins | **Cook Time:** 12-15 mins per batch | **Servings:** 12-15 cookies!

Why It's Essential: This cookie offers a unique and satisfying combination of pumpkin, warm spices, and the satisfying crunch of pumpkin seeds. Perfect for autumn snacking!

Ingredients:

- 1/2 cup sourdough discard (brown rice or sorghum starter is ideal)
- 1/4 cup pumpkin puree
- 1/4 cup pumpkin seeds
- 1/4 cup ground flaxseeds
- 1/4 teaspoon cinnamon
- 1/8 teaspoon ground ginger
- 1/8 teaspoon ground nutmeg
- 1 tablespoon molasses (or maple syrup)
- 1 large egg
- Pinch of salt

Alternative Ingredients:

- Swap pumpkin seeds for sunflower seeds or chopped walnuts.

Step-by-Step Instructions:

1. **Combine Ingredients:** In a bowl, mix sourdough discard, pumpkin puree, pumpkin seeds, flaxseeds, spices, molasses, egg, and salt.
2. **Chill (Optional):** For thicker cookies, chill the dough for 30 minutes.
3. **Shape & Bake:** Preheat oven to 350°F (175°C). Drop rounded tablespoons of dough onto a baking sheet lined with parchment paper. Bake for 12-15 minutes or until golden brown around the edges.
4. **Cool:** Let cookies cool on the baking sheet for a few minutes before transferring to a wire rack to cool completely.

Nutritional Values (per cookie):

- Calories: 100
- Carbohydrates: 9g
- Protein: 4g
- Fat: 6g
- Sodium: 40mg
- Fiber: 2g

Cooking Tips:

- Use unsweetened pumpkin puree for the best flavor balance.
- Toast the pumpkin seeds before adding them to the dough for extra flavor.

Special Diets:

- **Vegan:** Substitute the egg with a flax egg (1 tablespoon ground flaxseed + 3 tablespoons water).

Recipe 21: Banana Chia Bites

Prep Time: 10 mins | **Cook Time:** 12-15 mins per batch | **Servings:** 12-15 cookies

Why It's Essential: This cookie offers a naturally sweet treat packed with healthy fats from chia seeds, fiber from oats, and the subtle tang of sourdough.

Ingredients:

- 1 ripe banana, mashed.
- 1/4 cup sourdough discard (any variety)
- 1/4 cup chia seeds
- 1/4 cup rolled oats.
- 1 tablespoon honey or maple syrup
- 1/2 teaspoon cinnamon
- Pinch of salt

Alternative Ingredients:

- Add chopped nuts or dried fruit for extra texture and flavor.

Step-by-Step Instructions:

1. **Combine Ingredients:** In a bowl, mix mashed banana, sourdough discard, chia seeds, oats, honey or maple syrup, cinnamon, and salt.
2. **Chill:** Chill the dough in the refrigerator for at least 30 minutes to allow the chia seeds to soften and the dough to firm up.
3. **Shape & Bake:** Preheat oven to 350°F (175°C). Drop rounded tablespoons of dough onto a baking sheet lined with parchment paper. Bake for 12-15 minutes or until lightly golden brown.
4. **Cool:** Let cookies cool on the baking sheet before enjoying them or transferring them to an airtight container for storage.

Nutritional Values (per cookie):

- ❖ Calories: 70
- ❖ Carbohydrates: 10g
- ❖ Protein: 2g
- ❖ Fat: 3g
- ❖ Sodium: 15mg
- ❖ Fiber: 2g

Cooking Tips:

- ✓ Use a very ripe banana for optimal sweetness and easy mashing.
- ✓ For a more decadent treat, add a sprinkle of chocolate chips to the dough.

Special Diets:

- **Vegan**: This recipe is already vegan-friendly!

Recipe 22: PB & J Swirl

Prep Time: 10 mins | **Cook Time:** 12-15 mins per batch | **Servings:** 12-15 cookies

Why It's Essential: This cookie combines the classic flavor combo of peanut butter and jelly with the unique tang of sourdough for a fun and satisfying treat.

Ingredients:

- 1/2 cup sourdough discard (any variety)
- 1/4 cup peanut butter (creamy or chunky)
- 1/4 cup mashed raspberries (fresh or frozen, thawed, and drained)
- 1/4 cup almond flour
- 1 large egg
- 1 tablespoon honey or maple syrup
- 1/4 teaspoon baking soda
- Pinch of salt

Alternative Ingredients:

- Swap peanut butter for your favorite nut or seed butter.
- Use a different type of berry (e.g., blueberries, strawberries) for the swirl.

Step-by-Step Instructions:

1. **Combine Ingredients:** In a bowl, mix sourdough discard, peanut butter, mashed raspberries, almond flour, egg, honey or maple syrup, baking soda, and salt.
2. **Shape & Bake:** Preheat oven to 350°F (175°C). Drop rounded tablespoons of dough onto a baking sheet lined with parchment paper. Use a spoon or your finger to create a slight indentation in the middle of each cookie.
3. **Add Swirl:** Fill the indentations with a small dollop of your favorite jam or jelly.
4. **Bake:** Bake for 12-15 minutes or until golden brown around the edges.
5. **Cool:** Let cookies cool on the baking sheet for a few minutes before transferring to a wire rack to cool completely.

Nutritional Values (per cookie):

- Calories: 110
- Carbohydrates: 9g
- Protein: 5g
- Fat: 7g
- Sodium: 60mg
- Fiber: 2g

Cooking Tips:

- Use natural peanut butter (or your chosen nut butter) for the best flavor.
- Don't overfill the indentations, as the jam or jelly may spread during baking.

Special Diets:

- **Vegan**: Substitute the egg with a flax egg (1 tablespoon ground flaxseed + 3 tablespoons water). Ensure your jam or jelly is vegan.

Recipe 23: Blueberry Lemon Zest

Prep Time: 10 mins | **Cook Time:** 12-15 mins per batch | **Servings:** 12-15 cookies

Why It's Essential: This cookie offers a delightful combination of sweet blueberries and the bright, citrusy tang of lemon zest with the unique flavor of sourdough.

Ingredients:

- 1/2 cup sourdough discard (any variety)
- 1/2 cup mashed blueberries (fresh or frozen)
- 1/2 cup almond flour
- 1 teaspoon lemon zest
- 1 large egg
- 2 tablespoons honey or maple syrup
- 1/4 teaspoon baking soda
- Pinch of salt

Alternative Ingredients:

- Swap blueberries with raspberries or chopped strawberries.

Step-by-Step Instructions:

1. **Combine Ingredients:** In a bowl, mix sourdough discard, mashed blueberries, almond flour, lemon zest, egg, honey or maple syrup, baking soda, and salt.
2. **Shape & Bake:** Preheat oven to 350°F (175°C). Drop rounded tablespoons of dough onto a baking sheet lined with parchment paper.
3. **Bake:** Bake for 12-15 minutes or until golden brown around the edges.
4. **Cool:** Let cookies cool on the baking sheet for a few minutes before transferring to a wire rack to cool completely.

Nutritional Values (per cookie):

- Calories: 80
- Carbohydrates: 9g
- Protein: 4g
- Fat: 4g
- Sodium: 30mg
- Fiber: 2g

Cooking Tips:

- ✓ If using frozen blueberries, thaw and drain them before adding to the dough.
- ✓ For an extra burst of lemon flavor, drizzle a light lemon glaze over the cooled cookies.

Special Diets:

- **Vegan**: Substitute the egg with a flax egg (1 tablespoon ground flaxseed + 3 tablespoons water).

Recipe 24: Tropical Coconut Bites

Prep Time: 10 mins | **Cook Time:** 12-15 mins per batch | **Servings:** 12-15 cookies

Why It's Essential: This cookie offers a delightful mix of textures with shredded coconut and diced pineapple, with a hint of sweetness and the unique tang of sourdough for a taste of paradise.

Ingredients:

- 1/2 cup sourdough discard (millet or amaranth starter complements the tropical flavors)
- 1/4 cup shredded coconut
- 1/4 cup finely diced pineapple (fresh or canned, well-drained)
- 1/4 cup ground macadamia nuts (or almonds)
- 1 tablespoon honey or maple syrup
- 1 large egg
- Pinch of salt

Alternative Ingredients:

- Swap pineapple for diced mango or papaya.

Step-by-Step Instructions:

1. **Combine Ingredients:** In a bowl, mix sourdough discard, shredded coconut, diced pineapple, ground nuts, honey or maple syrup, egg, and salt.
2. **Shape & Bake:** Preheat oven to 350°F (175°C). Drop rounded tablespoons of dough onto a baking sheet lined with parchment paper.
3. **Bake:** Bake for 12-15 minutes or until golden brown and slightly puffed.
4. **Cool:** Let cookies cool on the baking sheet for a few minutes before transferring to a wire rack to cool completely.

Nutritional Values (per cookie):

- ❖ Calories: 100
- ❖ Carbohydrates: 9g
- ❖ Protein: 4g
- ❖ Fat: 6g
- ❖ Sodium: 20mg
- ❖ Fiber: 2g

Cooking Tips:

- ✓ Use unsweetened shredded coconut for the best flavor balance.
- ✓ Finely dice the pineapple for even distribution within the cookies.

Special Diets:

- **Vegan**: Substitute the egg with a flax egg (1 tablespoon ground flaxseed + 3 tablespoons water).

Recipe 25: Tropical Coconut Bites

Prep Time: 10 mins | **Cook Time:** 12-15 mins per batch | **Servings:** 12-15 cookies

Why It's Essential: This cookie offers a delightful mix of textures with shredded coconut and diced pineapple, with a hint of sweetness and the unique tang of sourdough for a taste of paradise.

Ingredients:

- 1/2 cup sourdough discard (millet or amaranth starter complements the tropical flavors)
- 1/4 cup shredded coconut
- 1/4 cup finely diced pineapple (fresh or canned, well-drained)
- 1/4 cup ground macadamia nuts (or almonds)
- 1 tablespoon honey or maple syrup
- 1 large egg
- Pinch of salt

Alternative Ingredients:

Swap pineapple for diced mango or papaya.

Step-by-Step Instructions:

1. **Combine Ingredients:** In a bowl, mix sourdough discard, shredded coconut, diced pineapple, ground nuts, honey or maple syrup, egg, and salt.
2. **Shape & Bake:** Preheat oven to 350°F (175°C). Drop rounded tablespoons of dough onto a baking sheet lined with parchment paper.
3. **Bake:** Bake for 12-15 minutes or until golden brown and slightly puffed.
4. **Cool:** Let cookies cool on the baking sheet for a few minutes before transferring to a wire rack to cool completely.

Nutritional Values (per cookie):

- Calories: 100
- Carbohydrates: 9g
- Protein: 4g
- Fat: 6g
- Sodium: 20mg
- Fiber: 2g

Cooking Tips:

- Use unsweetened shredded coconut for the best flavor balance.
- Finely dice the pineapple for even distribution within the cookies.

Special Diets:

- **Vegan:** Substitute the egg with a flax egg (1 tablespoon ground flaxseed + 3 tablespoons water).

Recipe 26: Double Chocolate Delight

Prep Time: 10 mins | **Cook Time:** 12-15 mins per batch | **Servings:** 12-15 cookies

Why It's Essential: This decadent cookie is perfect for any chocolate lover! The combination of unsweetened cocoa powder and chocolate chips delivers a rich chocolate flavor, complemented by the subtle sourdough tang.

Ingredients:

- 1/2 cup sourdough discard (any variety works well)
- 1/2 cup almond flour
- 1/4 cup unsweetened cocoa powder
- 1/2 cup chocolate chips (dark, semi-sweet, or a mixture)
- 1 large egg
- 1 tablespoon maple syrup
- 1/4 teaspoon baking soda
- Pinch of salt

Alternative Ingredients:

- Swap almond flour with another gluten-free flour blend.
- Use chopped dark chocolate instead of chocolate chips for an even more intense chocolate flavor.

Step-by-Step Instructions:

1. **Combine Ingredients:** In a bowl, mix sourdough discard, almond flour, cocoa powder, chocolate chips, egg, maple syrup, baking soda, and salt.
2. **Chill (Optional):** For thicker cookies, chill the dough for 30 minutes.
3. **Shape & Bake:** Preheat oven to 350°F (175°C). Drop rounded tablespoons of dough onto a baking sheet lined with parchment paper.
4. **Bake:** Bake for 12-15 minutes or until golden brown around the edges and the centers are slightly set.
5. **Cool:** Let cookies cool on the baking sheet for a few minutes before transferring to a wire rack to cool completely.

Nutritional Values (per cookie):

- Calories: 130
- Carbohydrates: 11g
- Protein: 4g
- Fat: 8g
- Sodium: 40mg
- Fiber: 2g

Cooking Tips:

- ✓ Use high-quality cocoa powder for the best chocolate flavor.
- ✓ Sprinkle a pinch of sea salt on top of the cookies before baking for a sweet and salty flavor contrast.

Special Diets:

- **Vegan:** Substitute the egg with a flax egg (1 tablespoon ground flaxseed + 3 tablespoons water). Ensure your chocolate chips are dairy-free.
- **Gluten-free:** This recipe is already gluten-free!

Chapter 8: Savory Sensations: Crackers & Crostini (7 Recipes)

Dive into the delightful world of savory snacks with our chapter on "Crackers & Crostini." This collection of seven recipes offers an array of crisp, flavorful options that are perfect for any occasion, whether it's a casual family gathering, an elegant cocktail party, or a relaxing evening at home.

In this chapter, we celebrate the art of baking with recipes that transform simple ingredients into extraordinary snacks. Each recipe is crafted to bring out the unique flavors and textures of homemade crackers and crostini, ensuring that your appetizer tray is anything but ordinary.

We'll guide you through the process of crafting crackers that are both crispy and rich in flavor, with variations that include everything from seeded multigrain to spicy pepper and cheese-infused delights. Additionally, you'll learn how to make crostini, the perfect base for a variety of toppings, from classic bruschetta to sophisticated spreads and everything in between.

These recipes not only focus on taste but also on the joy of creating something from scratch. You'll find detailed instructions on how to achieve the perfect crunch, tips for flavor combinations, and ideas for using these crackers and crostini as part of larger dishes or as standalone snacks.

Moreover, we'll explore how these homemade creations can be healthier alternatives to store-bought options, free from unnecessary preservatives and customizable to fit dietary needs and preferences.

Get ready to roll out dough, sprinkle seeds, and experiment with seasonings as we delve into the satisfying process of baking your own crackers and crostini. This chapter promises to equip you with all you need to whip up impressive, delicious, and versatile snacks that are sure to wow your guests and satisfy your savory cravings.

Let's get baking and bring some crunch to your culinary repertoire!

Recipe 27: Seeded Powerhouse Crackers: Combine sourdough discard (sorghum or brown rice starter), ground flaxseeds, sunflower seeds, chia seeds, herbs, and a touch of olive oil. Roll thinly, score, and bake until crispy.

Recipe 28: Chickpea & Herb Surprise: Blend sourdough discard, cooked chickpeas, herbs (rosemary, thyme), garlic powder, a touch of olive oil, and a sprinkle of nutritional yeast for cheesy flavor. Spread thinly, score, and bake.

Recipe 29: Zesty Parmesan & Almond: Mix sourdough discard, finely grated parmesan cheese, almond flour, dried herbs, a hint of garlic, and a touch of olive oil. Pat into shapes and bake until golden brown.

Recipe 30: Spiced Lentil & Quinoa: Combine sourdough discard, cooked red lentils, cooked quinoa, spices (cumin, coriander), finely chopped onion, and a hint of chili flakes. Form into cracker shapes and bake for a crisp and flavorful snack.

Recipe 31: Everything Bagel Crostini: Slice gluten-free sourdough bread thinly. Toss with olive oil, a sprinkle of sourdough discard, and "everything bagel" seasoning (poppy seeds, sesame seeds, dried onion, garlic, etc.). Bake until crisp.

Recipe 32: Smoky Paprika & Chickpea: Combine sourdough discard, mashed chickpeas, smoked paprika, garlic powder, herbs, and a touch of olive oil. Spread on thin slices of gluten-free bread and bake until golden.

Recipe 33: Mediterranean Olive & Feta Crumble: Top thin slices of gluten-free sourdough bread with olive tapenade, crumbled feta cheese, a sprinkle of dried oregano, and a drizzle of sourdough discard. Broil until bubbly and slightly browned.

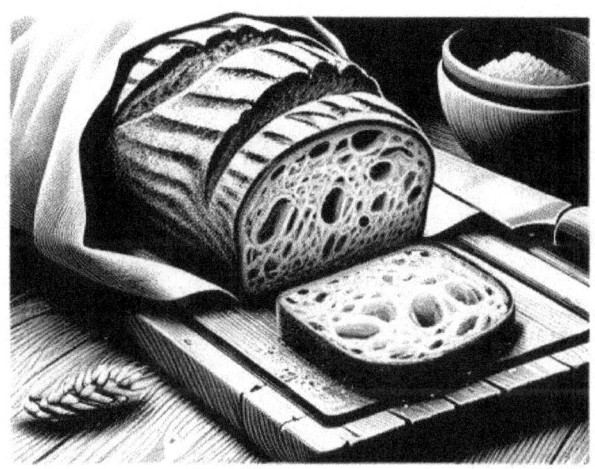

Watch the Dough, Not the Clock: "Focus on the dough's volume, texture, and responsiveness to touch to determine readiness, rather than adhering strictly to timing."

Recipe 27: Seeded Powerhouse Crackers

Prep Time: 15 mins | **Cook Time:** 20-25 mins | **Servings:** Depends on cracker size

Why It's Essential: These crackers offer a satisfying crunch, healthy fats, protein, and fiber from the seeds, and a subtle tang from the sourdough.

Ingredients:

- 1 cup sourdough discard (brown rice or sorghum starter is ideal)
- 1/4 cup ground flaxseeds
- 1/4 cup sunflower seeds
- 1/4 cup chia seeds
- 1 tablespoon dried herbs of choice (e.g., rosemary, thyme, oregano)
- 1 tablespoon olive oil
- 1/2 teaspoon salt
- 1/4 teaspoon black pepper

Alternative Ingredients:

- Swap some seeds for pumpkin seeds or sesame seeds.
- Add a pinch of chili powder or smoked paprika for a touch of spice.

Step-by-Step Instructions:

1. **Combine Ingredients:** In a bowl, mix sourdough discard, ground flaxseeds, sunflower seeds, chia seeds, dried herbs, olive oil, salt, and pepper.
2. **Roll & Score:** Roll the dough out very thinly (1/8-inch thickness) between two sheets of parchment paper. Score into desired cracker shapes with a knife or pizza cutter.
3. **Bake:** Transfer to a baking sheet lined with parchment paper. Bake in a preheated oven at 350°F (175°C) for 20-25 minutes or until golden brown and crispy.
4. **Cool & Break:** Let crackers cool completely on the baking sheet before breaking them apart along the scored lines.

Nutritional Values (per serving):

- ❖ Calories: 100
- ❖ Carbohydrates: 6g
- ❖ Protein: 5g
- ❖ Fat: 7g
- ❖ Sodium: 100mg
- ❖ Fiber: 3g

Cooking Tips:

- ✓ Roll the dough as thinly as possible for extra crisp crackers.
- ✓ If the dough is too sticky, add a touch of gluten-free flour.

Special Diets:

- **Vegan**: This recipe is already vegan-friendly!

Recipe 28: Chickpea & Herb Surprise

Prep Time: 15 mins | **Cook Time:** 20-25 mins | **Servings:** Depends on cracker size

Why It's Essential: This recipe offers a unique flavor combination, a protein boost from chickpeas, cheesy notes from the nutritional yeast, and the subtle tang of sourdough.

Ingredients:

- 1 cup sourdough discard (any variety)
- 1 cup cooked chickpeas, drained and rinsed.
- 1/4 cup chopped fresh herbs (rosemary, thyme, parsley, or a combination)
- 1 tablespoon garlic powder
- 1 tablespoon nutritional yeast
- 1 tablespoon olive oil
- 1/2 teaspoon salt
- 1/4 teaspoon black pepper

Alternative Ingredients:

- Swap cooked chickpeas for white beans or lentils.

Step-by-Step Instructions:

1. **Blend Ingredients:** In a food processor, combine sourdough discard, cooked chickpeas, herbs, garlic powder, nutritional yeast, olive oil, salt, and pepper. Blend until a mostly smooth spread is formed.
2. **Roll & Score:** Spread the mixture evenly and thinly (1/4-inch thickness) onto a baking sheet lined with parchment paper. Score into desired cracker shapes with a knife or pizza cutter.
3. **Bake:** Bake in a preheated oven at 350°F (175°C) for 20-25 minutes or until golden brown and crispy.
4. **Cool & Break:** Let crackers cool completely on the baking sheet before breaking them apart along the scored lines.

Nutritional Values (per serving):

- Calories: 120
- Carbohydrates: 10g
- Protein: 6g
- Fat: 7g
- Sodium: 120mg
- Fiber: 4g

Cooking Tips:

- Adjust the consistency by adding a touch of water to the mixture for easier spreading.
- Top with a sprinkle of sesame seeds or poppy seeds before baking for extra flavor.

Special Diets:

- **Vegan:** This recipe is already vegan-friendly!

Recipe 29: Zesty Parmesan & Almond

Prep Time: 10 mins | **Cook Time:** 15-20 mins | **Servings:** Depends on cracker size

Why It's Essential: These crackers offer a savory and satisfying flavor with a hint of nutty richness from the almond flour and cheesy flavor from the parmesan.

Ingredients:

- 1 cup sourdough discard (any variety)
- 1/2 cup finely grated parmesan cheese.
- 1/2 cup almond flour
- 1 tablespoon dried herbs (Italian herbs, oregano, etc.)
- 1 teaspoon garlic powder
- 1 tablespoon olive oil
- 1/4 teaspoon salt
- 1/4 teaspoon black pepper

Step-by-Step Instructions:

1. **Combine Ingredients:** In a bowl, mix sourdough discard, parmesan cheese, almond flour, dried herbs, garlic powder, olive oil, salt, and pepper.
2. **Pat & Bake:** Pat the dough into a rectangle (around 1/4 inch thick) on a baking sheet lined with parchment paper. Bake in a preheated oven at 375°F (190°C) for 15-20 minutes or until golden brown.
3. **Cool & Break:** Let crackers cool completely on the baking sheet before breaking them into desired shapes.

Nutritional Values (per serving):

- ❖ Calories: 130
- ❖ Carbohydrates: 5g
- ❖ Protein: 8g
- ❖ Fat: 9g
- ❖ Sodium: 150mg
- ❖ Fiber: 2g

Cooking Tips:

✓ For a finer texture, pulse the almond flour in a food processor before adding it to the dough.

Special Diets:

- **Vegetarian:** This recipe is already vegetarian-friendly!

Recipe 30: Spiced Lentil & Quinoa

Prep Time: 20 mins (+ lentil & quinoa cooking time) | **Cook Time:** 20-25 mins | **Servings:** Depends on cracker size

Why It's Essential: This recipe offers a unique combination of flavors and textures, with protein and fiber from the lentils and quinoa and a delightful warmth from the spices.

Ingredients:

- 1 cup sourdough discard (brown rice or sorghum starter is ideal)
- 1/2 cup cooked red lentils.
- 1/2 cup cooked quinoa
- 1/4 cup finely chopped onion.
- 1 teaspoon cumin
- 1/2 teaspoon coriander powder
- 1/4 teaspoon chili flakes (optional)
- 2 tablespoons olive oil
- 1/2 teaspoon salt
- 1/4 teaspoon black pepper

Alternative Ingredients:

- Use other types of lentils (green, brown) or swap them for beans.

Step-by-Step Instructions:

1. **Combine Ingredients:** In a bowl, gently mash the cooked lentils and mix with sourdough discard, quinoa, chopped onion, spices, olive oil, salt, and pepper.
2. **Roll & Score:** Spread the mixture evenly and thinly (1/4-inch thickness) onto a baking sheet lined with parchment paper. Score into desired cracker shapes with a knife or pizza cutter.
3. **Bake:** Bake in a preheated oven at 350°F (175°C) for 20-25 minutes or until golden brown and crispy.
4. **Cool & Break:** Let crackers cool completely on the baking sheet before breaking them apart along the scored lines.

Nutritional Values (per serving):

- Calories: 150
- Carbohydrates: 15g
- Protein: 8g
- Fat: 7g
- Sodium: 130mg
- Fiber: 5g

Cooking Tips:

- ✓ Don't overcook the lentils; they should be tender but still hold their shape.
- ✓ If the mixture feels too wet, add a touch of gluten-free flour.

Special Diets:

- **Vegan:** This recipe is already vegan-friendly!

Recipe 31: Everything Bagel Crostini

Prep Time: 10 mins | **Cook Time:** 15-20 mins | **Servings:** Depends on bread slices used

Why It's Essential: This recipe brings the beloved flavor of "everything bagels" to a satisfying, crispy crostini. Perfect for dips, spreads, or toppings.

Ingredients:

- 6-8 slices of slightly stale gluten-free sourdough bread
- 2 tablespoons olive oil
- 1 tablespoon sourdough discard (any variety)
- 1 tablespoon "Everything Bagel" seasoning (poppy seeds, sesame seeds, dried onion, garlic flakes, salt)

Step-by-Step Instructions:

1. **Slice & Toss:** Cut the bread into thin slices. In a bowl, toss the bread slices with olive oil, sourdough discard, and "everything bagel" seasoning.
2. **Bake:** Spread the slices in a single layer on a baking sheet. Bake in a preheated oven at 375°F (190°C) for 15-20 minutes or until golden brown and crisp.
3. **Cool:** Let the crostini cool completely on the baking sheet before serving or storing.

Nutritional Values (per serving):

- Calories: 140
- Carbohydrates: 10g
- Protein: 4g
- Fat: 10g
- Sodium: 150mg (varies depending on "everything bagel" seasoning)
- Fiber: 2g

Cooking Tips:

- ✓ Use slightly stale bread for the best crispy texture.
- ✓ Adjust the amount of "everything bagel" seasoning according to your preference.

Special Diets:

- **Vegan**: Use a plant-based sourdough discard. Ensure your "everything bagel" seasoning is vegan-friendly.

Recipe 32: Smoky Paprika & Chickpea

Prep Time: 15 mins | **Cook Time:** 15-20 mins | **Servings:** Depends on bread slices used

Why It's Essential: This recipe offers a warm, smoky flavor with a protein boost from the chickpeas and a satisfying savory element perfect for a variety of toppings.

Ingredients:

- 6-8 slices of slightly stale gluten-free sourdough bread
- 1 cup cooked chickpeas, drained and rinsed.
- 1 tablespoon olive oil
- 1 teaspoon smoked paprika.
- 1/2 teaspoon garlic powder
- 1/4 teaspoon dried herbs (thyme, oregano, etc.)
- 1 tablespoon sourdough discard (any variety)
- 1/4 teaspoon salt
- 1/4 teaspoon black pepper

Alternative Ingredients:

- Substitute chickpeas with another type of cooked bean.

Step-by-Step Instructions:

1. **Mash & Season:** In a bowl, lightly mash the chickpeas with a fork. Add olive oil, smoked paprika, garlic powder, herbs, sourdough discard, salt, and pepper. Mix well.
2. **Top & Bake:** Spread the chickpea mixture evenly on the bread slices. Bake in a preheated oven at 375°F (190°C) for 15-20 minutes or until golden brown and crisp.
3. **Cool:** Let the crostini cool slightly before serving or storing.

Nutritional Values (per serving):

- Calories: 170
- Carbohydrates: 15g
- Protein: 8g
- Fat: 10g
- Sodium: 180mg
- Fiber: 5g

Cooking Tips:

- ✓ Adjust the level of spiciness by adding a pinch of cayenne pepper or red pepper flakes.
- ✓ Top with a sprinkle of fresh parsley or cilantro for a pop of color and freshness.

Special Diets:

- **Vegan:** This recipe is already vegan-friendly!

Recipe 33: Mediterranean Olive & Feta Crumble

Prep Time: 10 mins | **Cook Time:** 5-8 mins (Broiling) | **Servings:** Depends on bread slices used

Why It's Essential: This crostino offers a burst of fresh, tangy Mediterranean flavors with the combination of olives, feta, and the subtle brightness of sourdough.

Ingredients:

- 6-8 slices of slightly stale gluten-free sourdough bread
- 1/4 cup olive tapenade
- 1/4 cup crumbled feta cheese
- 1 teaspoon dried oregano
- 1 tablespoon sourdough discard (any variety)

Alternative Ingredients:

- Use other briny olives like kalamata in place of the olive tapenade.
- Substitute feta cheese with goat cheese.

Step-by-Step Instructions:

1. **Top & Drizzle:** Spread olive tapenade evenly over the bread slices. Crumble feta cheese over the tapenade, sprinkle with dried oregano, and finish with a drizzle of sourdough discard.
2. **Broil:** Place the crostini on a baking sheet and broil for 5-8 minutes, or until the feta is slightly melted and bubbly and the edges are golden brown.
3. **Serve:** Serve immediately while warm and melty.

Nutritional Values (per serving):

- Calories: 160
- Carbohydrates: 10g
- Protein: 6g
- Fat: 12g
- Sodium: 350mg
- Fiber: 2g

Cooking Tips:

- ✓ Watch the crostini carefully while broiling to prevent burning.
- ✓ Add a sprinkle of fresh lemon zest or chopped herbs for extra flavor.

Special Diets:

- **Vegetarian**: This recipe is already vegetarian-friendly!

Chapter 9: Breadcrumbs (5 Recipes + Uses)

In this innovative chapter, we explore the versatility and culinary potential of breadcrumbs made from gluten-free sourdough bread. Breadcrumbs are a staple in kitchens worldwide, used to add texture and flavor to a myriad of dishes. Here, we present five unique recipes that not only enhance meals but also provide creative ways to use up leftover sourdough bread, embracing a zero-waste approach to cooking.

Each recipe in this chapter transforms stale gluten-free sourdough bread into something spectacular. From classic herbed breadcrumbs perfect for topping casseroles and vegetables to protein-packed versions ideal for creating a crunchy coating on meats, these recipes are designed to be easy, flavorful, and versatile. We also introduce innovative combinations like spiced Panko-style breadcrumbs for those who love a crispy finish and a quinoa and almond mixture that offers a nutritious twist to traditional uses.

Beyond the recipes, this chapter dives into the practical uses of each type of breadcrumb, providing you with the inspiration to enhance your cooking routines. You'll learn how breadcrumbs can be used to bind, coat, or sprinkle over dishes for added crunch and flavor. Each recipe is accompanied by tips on how to best incorporate these breadcrumbs into everyday meals and special occasion dishes alike.

Whether you're looking to craft a perfect crusty topping for a baked dish or need a robust binder for patties and loaves, these gluten-free sourdough breadcrumbs offer something for every chef's need.

Let's reduce waste and increase taste as we explore the delightful versatility of sourdough breadcrumbs!

1. **Classic Herbed Breadcrumbs:** Toast stale GF sourdough bread blended into crumbs with sourdough discard, herbs de Provence, garlic powder, and a touch of olive oil. Uses: Topping casseroles, fish, or roasted vegetables.

2. **Protein-Packed Breadcrumbs:** Grind toasted GF sourdough bread with sunflower seeds, pumpkin seeds, nutritional yeast, herbs, and a touch of olive oil. Excellent for breaded chicken or fish.

3. **Spiced Panko-Style:** Pulse stale GF sourdough into large crumbs, mix with sourdough discard, paprika, garlic powder, dried oregano, and a touch of oil. Perfect for crispy coatings.

4. **Quinoa & Almond Crumbs:** Combine ground GF sourdough bread, cooked quinoa, grated parmesan, finely chopped almonds, herbs, and a touch of olive oil. Great for veggie burgers or meatloaf.

5. **Lemony Herb Breadcrumbs:** Process toasted GF sourdough, lemon zest, fresh parsley, dried basil, garlic powder, and a touch of olive oil. Ideal for a flavorful crust on baked fish.

Recipe 34: Classic Herbed Breadcrumbs

Prep Time: 10 mins | **Cook Time:** 5-10 mins (toasting) | **Yield:** Depends on the bread used

Why It's Essential: This recipe offers a classic take on breadcrumbs packed with herby freshness. Perfect as a versatile topping or breading for a variety of dishes.

Ingredients:

- 2-3 cups stale gluten-free sourdough bread (brown rice or sorghum starter is preferable as they add a neutral flavor base)
- 1 tablespoon sourdough discard (any variety)
- 1 tablespoon dried herbs de Provence (or use your favorite herby mix)
- 1/2 teaspoon garlic powder
- 1 tablespoon olive oil
- Pinch of salt and black pepper

Step-by-Step Instructions:

1. **Toast Bread:** Tear the stale sourdough bread into smaller pieces. Toast in a preheated oven at 350°F (175°C) for 5-10 minutes or until lightly browned and crisp.
2. **Pulse into Crumbs:** Pulse the toasted bread in a food processor into coarse crumbs.
3. **Add Seasonings:** Mix in the sourdough discard, herbs de Provence, garlic powder, olive oil, salt, and pepper.

Uses:

- Topping for casseroles, mac & cheese, and roasted vegetables.
- Breading for fish or chicken cutlets.
- Mix into meatballs or meatloaf for extra texture.

Nutritional Values (per 1/4 cup serving):

- Calories: 80
- Carbohydrates: 10g
- Protein: 2g
- Fat: 4g
- Sodium: 80mg
- Fiber: 2g

Cooking Tips:

- Adjust the herbs to your liking.
- If you don't have stale bread, dry fresh bread slices in a low oven until crisp.

Special Diets:

- **Vegan:** Use a plant-based sourdough discard.

Recipe 35: Protein-Packed Breadcrumbs

Prep Time: 10 mins | **Cook Time:** 5-10 mins (toasting) | **Yield:** Depends on the bread used

Why It's Essential: This recipe adds extra protein and healthy fats from seeds and nutritional yeast — perfect for boosting the nutritional value of breaded dishes.

Ingredients:

- 2-3 cups stale gluten-free sourdough bread (brown rice or sorghum starter is preferable as they add a neutral flavor base)
- 1/4 cup sunflower seeds
- 1/4 cup pumpkin seeds
- 2 tablespoons nutritional yeast
- 1 tablespoon dried herbs (Italian herbs, oregano, etc.)
- 1/2 teaspoon garlic powder
- 1 tablespoon olive oil
- Pinch of salt and black pepper

Step-by-Step Instructions:

1. **Toast Bread & Seeds:** Tear the stale sourdough bread into smaller pieces. Toast the bread and seeds together in a preheated oven at 350°F (175°C) for 5-10 minutes or until lightly browned and crisp.
2. **Grind into Crumbs:** Grind the toasted bread and seeds in a food processor into coarse crumbs.
3. **Add Seasonings:** Mix in nutritional yeast, dried herbs, garlic powder, olive oil, salt, and pepper.

Uses:

- Perfect for breaded chicken, fish, or tofu for a protein and nutrient boost.
- Great for adding a savory, crunchy topping to vegetables.

Nutritional Values (per 1/4 cup serving):

- Calories: 100
- Carbohydrates: 8g
- Protein: 5g
- Fat: 6g
- Sodium: 90mg
- Fiber: 2g

Cooking Tips:

- Add other seeds or nuts for extra flavor and crunch.
- Swap nutritional yeast for finely grated parmesan cheese (not vegan-friendly).

Special Diets:

- **Vegan**: This recipe is already vegan-friendly!

Recipe 36: Spiced Panko-Style

Prep Time: 10 mins | **Cook Time:** 5-10 mins (toasting) | **Yield:** Depends on the bread used

Why It's Essential: This recipe offers a larger, crunchier crumb similar to panko breadcrumbs. It is perfect for achieving a crisp texture in fried or baked dishes.

Ingredients:

- 2-3 cups stale gluten-free sourdough bread (a lighter crumbed bread works well)
- 1 tablespoon sourdough discard (any variety)
- 1 teaspoon smoked paprika (or regular paprika)
- 1/2 teaspoon garlic powder
- 1/2 teaspoon dried oregano
- 1 tablespoon olive oil
- Pinch of salt and black pepper

Step-by-Step Instructions:

1. **Pulse into Large Crumbs:** Tear the stale sourdough bread into larger pieces. Pulse in a food processor into coarse, panko-like crumbs (avoid over-processing).
2. **Add Seasonings:** Mix in smoked paprika, garlic powder, oregano, sourdough discard, olive oil, salt, and pepper.

Uses:

- Ideal for a super crispy coating on baked or fried chicken, fish, or vegetables.
- Use as a crunchy topping for casseroles or mac & cheese.

Nutritional Values (per 1/4 cup serving):

- Calories: 90
- Carbohydrates: 10g
- Protein: 2g
- Fat: 5g
- Sodium: 90mg
- Fiber: 2g

Cooking Tips:

- Adjust the spices to your liking – get creative!
- For extra crispness, spread the crumbs in a single layer on a baking sheet and bake at a low temperature (250°F/120°C) for a few minutes to dry them out further.

Special Diets:

- **Vegan**: Use a plant-based sourdough discard.

Recipe 37: Quinoa & Almond Crumbs

Prep Time: 15 mins (+ quinoa cooking time) | **Cook Time:** 5-10 mins (toasting) | **Yield:** Depends on the bread used

Why It's Essential: This recipe offers a unique texture and nutty flavor due to the addition of quinoa and almonds, along with a boost of protein and healthy fats.

Ingredients:

- 2-3 cups stale gluten-free sourdough bread (brown rice or sorghum starter works well)
- 1/2 cup cooked quinoa
- 1/4 cup grated parmesan cheese.
- 1/4 cup finely chopped almonds.
- 1 tablespoon dried herbs (Italian herbs, chives, etc.)
- 1 tablespoon olive oil
- Pinch of salt and black pepper

Step-by-Step Instructions:

1. **Toast-Bread:** Tear the stale sourdough bread into smaller pieces. Toast in a preheated oven at 350°F (175°C) for 5-10 minutes or until lightly browned and crisp.
2. **Grind into Crumbs:** Grind the toasted bread, cooked quinoa, almonds, and parmesan cheese in a food processor into coarse crumbs.
3. **Add Seasonings:** Mix in dried herbs, olive oil, salt, and pepper.

Uses:

- Excellent for adding to meatballs or meatloaf for added flavor and texture.
- Perfect for a flavorful and crunchy topping on baked vegetables.

Nutritional Values (per 1/4 cup serving):

- ❖ Calories: 130
- ❖ Carbohydrates: 10g
- ❖ Protein: 7g
- ❖ Fat: 7g
- ❖ Sodium: 120mg
- ❖ Fiber: 3g

Cooking Tips:

- ✓ Use pre-cooked, cooled quinoa for convenience.
- ✓ Add other nuts or seeds for an additional flavor boost.

Special Diets:

- **Vegetarian**: This recipe is already vegetarian-friendly!

Recipe 38: Lemony Herb Breadcrumbs

Prep Time: 10 mins | **Cook Time:** 5-10 mins (toasting) | **Yield:** Depends on the bread used

Why It's Essential: This recipe offers a burst of fresh, citrusy flavor perfect for enhancing fish and seafood dishes.

Ingredients:

- 2-3 cups stale gluten-free sourdough bread (a lighter crumbed bread works well)
- 1 tablespoon lemon zest
- 2 tablespoons chopped fresh parsley.
- 1 tablespoon dried basil
- 1/2 teaspoon garlic powder
- 1 tablespoon olive oil
- Pinch of salt and black pepper

Step-by-Step Instructions:

1. **Toast Bread:** Tear the stale sourdough bread into smaller pieces. Toast in a preheated oven at 350°F (175°C) for 5-10 minutes or until lightly browned and crisp.
2. **Grind into Crumbs:** Process the toasted bread with lemon zest, parsley, basil, garlic powder, olive oil, salt, and pepper in a food processor into coarse crumbs.

Uses:

- Ideal for a flavorful crust on baked or pan-fried fish.
- Sprinkle on top of roasted vegetables for a burst of flavor.

Nutritional Values (per 1/4 cup serving):

- Calories: 85
- Carbohydrates: 10g
- Protein: 2g
- Fat: 5g
- Sodium: 80mg
- Fiber: 2g

Cooking Tips:

✓ Use a combination of fresh herbs for a more vibrant flavor profile.

Special Diets:

- **Vegan**: Use a plant-based sourdough discard.

Chapter 10: Stuffing & Panzanella (6 Recipes)

Chapter 10 delves into the heartwarming world of comfort foods, focusing on two beloved dishes that turn bread into culinary stars: stuffing and Panzanella. This collection of six recipes explores the delightful versatility and satisfying textures of these dishes, making excellent use of sourdough bread to elevate flavors and add a rustic touch.

Stuffing, traditionally served alongside roasted meats, is not just for holiday tables. In this chapter, you'll discover how to prepare stuffing that is perfect for any occasion, whether you're looking to complement a weeknight roast or create a centerpiece for a festive meal. Each recipe is crafted to bring out the best in sourdough bread, using its unique tanginess to enhance the overall flavor profile of the stuffing.

On the other hand, Panzanella, a Tuscan salad made primarily of bread and tomatoes, showcases how stale bread can be transformed into a vibrant, fresh dish. Our recipes will guide you through making various panzanella versions that burst with seasonal ingredients and bold dressings, which are ideal for light lunches or as a side to any meal.

We'll cover:

Recipe 39: Quinoa, Kale, & Cranberry: Combine cubed GF sourdough bread, cooked quinoa, sautéed kale, dried cranberries, pecans, herbs, and a broth-based dressing with sourdough discard.

Recipe 40: Mediterranean Panzanella: Toss cubed GF sourdough bread with tomatoes, cucumbers, kalamata olives, red onion, fresh basil, a vinaigrette with sourdough discard, and crumbled feta cheese.

Recipe 41: Southwestern Black Bean & Corn: Combine cubed GF sourdough bread, cooked black beans, corn, diced bell peppers, cilantro, spices, and a lime/sourdough discard dressing.

Recipe 42: Lentil & Mushroom Stuffing: Sauteed mushrooms, onions, cooked lentils, herbs, GF sourdough bread cubes, vegetable broth, and sourdough discard. Rich and savory.

Recipe 43: Sausage & Apple Delight: Crumbled GF sausage, cubed GF sourdough bread, diced apple, celery, herbs, and a broth-based dressing with sourdough discard.

Recipe 44: Greek-Inspired Panzanella: Cubed GF sourdough bread, cherry tomatoes, cucumber, chickpeas, red onion, fresh oregano, and a red wine vinegar and sourdough discard dressing.

This chapter also includes practical tips on selecting the right type of sourdough for each recipe, preparation methods that maximize flavor absorption, and creative variations to customize dishes to your taste. Whether refreshing old favorites or discovering new ones, these recipes ensure your sourdough bread never goes to waste.

Prepare to be inspired as we turn humble ingredients into spectacular meals that comfort the soul and delight the senses. Let's dive into the art of transforming sourdough bread into stuffing and Panzanella that will enliven your table and your taste buds!

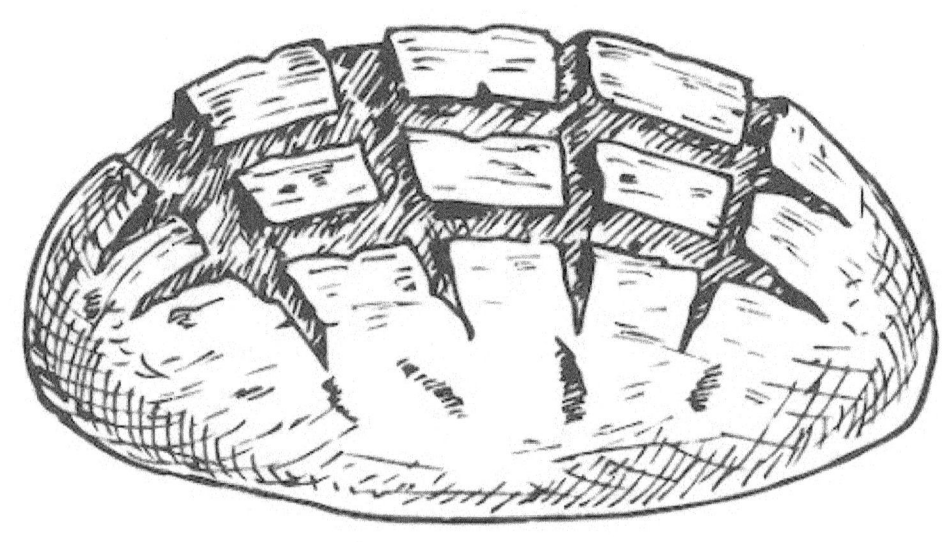

__Preheat Your Baking Vessel__: "Always preheat your Dutch oven or baking stone well before baking to mimic a professional oven environment, giving your sourdough a strong burst of initial heat."

Recipe 39: Quinoa, Kale & Cranberry

Prep Time: 20 mins (+ quinoa cooking time) | **Cook Time:** 15-20 mins (sautéing + baking) | **Servings:** 6-8

Why It's Essential: This recipe offers a balanced and nutritious stuffing or salad with a protein boost from quinoa, antioxidants from kale, and sweetness from cranberries.

Ingredients:

- 4-5 cups cubed gluten-free sourdough bread (brown rice or sorghum starter is ideal)
- 1 cup cooked quinoa
- 2 cups chopped kale.
- 1/2 cup dried cranberries
- 1/4 cup chopped pecans (or walnuts)
- 1 tablespoon olive oil
- 1/2 cup chopped onion.
- 1-2 cloves garlic, minced.
- 1 teaspoon dried sage or thyme
- 1/2 cup vegetable broth or chicken broth
- 1/4 cup sourdough discard (any variety)
- Salt and pepper to taste

Step-by-Step Instructions:

1. **Sauté:** Sauté onions and garlic in olive oil until softened. Add kale and cook until wilted. Season with salt and pepper.
2. **Combine:** In a large bowl, combine sourdough bread cubes, quinoa, cranberries, pecans, sautéed kale mixture, herbs, broth, and sourdough discard.
3. **Bake (Stuffing):** Transfer to a baking dish and bake at 350°F (175°C) for 15-20 mins, or until heated through and lightly browned.
4. **Serve (Panzanella):** Toss the mixture with a simple vinaigrette if serving as a panzanella salad.

Nutritional Values (per serving):

- ❖ Calories: 250
- ❖ Carbohydrates: 35g
- ❖ Protein: 10g
- ❖ Fat: 10g
- ❖ Sodium: 200mg
- ❖ Fiber: 6g

Cooking Tips:

- ✓ Add other dried fruits like apricots or cherries.
- ✓ Use pre-cooked or leftover quinoa for convenience.

Special Diets:

- **Vegan**: Use a plant-based broth and ensure your sourdough discard is plant-based.

Recipe 40: Mediterranean Panzanella

Prep Time: 15 mins | **Resting Time:** 15-30 mins | **Servings:** 4-6

Why It's Essential: This recipe features the classic Mediterranean flavors of tomatoes, cucumbers, olives, and feta, with the added tang of sourdough – perfect for a refreshing summer salad.

Ingredients:

- 4-5 cups cubed gluten-free sourdough bread (crusty bread works well)
- 2 cups cherry tomatoes halved or quartered.
- 1 cup chopped cucumber.
- 1/2 cup kalamata olives, pitted and halved.
- 1/4 cup chopped red onion.
- 1/4 cup fresh basil leaves roughly chopped.
- 1/4 cup crumbled feta cheese
- 3 tablespoons olive oil
- 2 tablespoons red wine vinegar
- 1 tablespoon sourdough discard (any variety)
- 1/2 teaspoon dried oregano
- Salt and pepper to taste

Alternative Ingredients:

- Swap cherry tomatoes for other types of tomatoes like heirloom or Roma.
- Substitute kalamata olives with other briny olives, like green olives.
- Use goat cheese or a vegan feta alternative if desired.

Step-by-Step Instructions:

1. **Toss Bread:** In a large bowl, combine sourdough bread cubes with a drizzle of olive oil and a pinch of salt.
2. **Make Dressing:** Whisk together the remaining olive oil, red wine vinegar, sourdough discard, oregano, salt, and pepper.
3. **Combine & Rest:** Add tomatoes, cucumbers, olives, onion, basil, feta (if using), and dressing to the bowl with the bread. Toss gently and let the salad rest for 15-30 minutes to allow the bread to soak up the flavors.
4. **Serve:** Taste and adjust seasoning with salt and pepper as needed. Serve immediately.
5. Nutritional Values (per serving):
- Calories: 280
- Carbohydrates: 30g
- Protein: 8g
- Fat: 18g
- Sodium: 400mg
- Fiber: 4g

Cooking Tips:

- ✓ Use stale bread for the best results in a panzanella.
- ✓ Add other Mediterranean-inspired ingredients like capers, artichoke hearts, or roasted bell peppers.

Special Diets:

- **Vegetarian**: This recipe is already vegetarian-friendly!
- **Vegan**: Use a plant-based sourdough; discard and substitute the feta cheese with a vegan alternative or omit.

Recipe 41: Southwestern Black Bean & Corn

Prep Time: 20 mins | **Cook Time:** 15-20 mins (sautéing/baking) | **Servings:** 6-8

Why It's Essential: This recipe offers a satisfying, hearty stuffing, or salad with a protein boost from black beans, sweetness from corn, and a touch of spice from chili powder.

Ingredients:

- 4-5 cups cubed gluten-free sourdough bread (brown rice or sorghum starter is ideal)
- 1 can (15 oz) black beans rinsed and drained.
- 1 cup corn kernels (fresh, frozen, or canned)
- 1/2 cup diced bell pepper (red, orange, or yellow)
- 1/4 cup chopped cilantro.
- 1 tablespoon olive oil
- 1/2 cup chopped onion.
- 1-2 cloves garlic, minced.
- 1 teaspoon chili powder
- 1/2 teaspoon cumin
- 1/2 cup vegetable broth or chicken broth
- 1/4 cup sourdough discard (any variety)
- 1/4 cup lime juice
- Salt and pepper to taste

Alternative Ingredients:

- Swap black beans for pinto beans or kidney beans.
- Add chopped jalapeño or a pinch of cayenne pepper for extra heat.

Step-by-Step Instructions:

1. **Sauté:** Sauté onions, garlic, and bell pepper in olive oil until softened. Season with salt and pepper. Add chili powder and cumin and cook for a minute more.
2. **Combine:** In a large bowl, combine sourdough bread cubes, black beans, corn, cilantro, sautéed vegetable mixture, broth, sourdough discard, lime juice, salt, and pepper.
3. **Bake (Stuffing):** Transfer to a baking dish and bake at 350°F (175°C) for 15-20 mins, or until heated through and lightly browned.
4. **Serve (Panzanella):** Toss with an additional drizzle of olive oil and lime juice if serving as a Panzanella salad.

Nutritional Values (per serving):

- Calories: 230
- Carbohydrates: 35g
- Protein: 9g
- Fat: 8g
- Sodium: 300mg
- Fiber: 7g

Cooking Tips:

- Add a sprinkle of shredded cheese (cheddar, Monterey Jack) on top before baking for a melty topping (not strictly Southwestern, but delicious!)
- Garnish with chopped avocado or a dollop of sour cream for an extra touch.

Special Diets:

- **Vegan**: Use a plant-based broth and ensure your sourdough discard is plant-based.
- **Vegetarian**: This recipe is already vegetarian-friendly.

Recipe 42: Lentil & Mushroom Stuffing

Prep Time: 20 mins (+ lentil cooking time) | **Cook Time:** 20-25 mins | **Servings:** 6-8

Why It's Essential: This hearty stuffing is packed with earthy flavors from mushrooms and lentils and protein for a satisfying vegetarian meal.

Ingredients:

- 4-5 cups cubed gluten-free sourdough bread (brown rice or sorghum starter is preferable)
- 1 cup cooked lentils (brown or green lentils work well)
- 8 ounces mushrooms, sliced.
- 1 tablespoon olive oil
- 1/2 cup chopped onion.
- 1-2 cloves garlic, minced.
- 1 tablespoon dried thyme or sage (or a mix of both)
- 1/2 cup vegetable broth or chicken broth
- 1/4 cup sourdough discard (any variety)
- Salt and pepper to taste

Alternative Ingredients:

- Use a variety of mushrooms like cremini, shiitake, or oyster mushrooms for deeper flavor.
- Substitute cooked lentils with other cooked beans like chickpeas.

Step-by-Step Instructions:

1. **Sauté:** Sauté onions and garlic in olive oil until softened. Add mushrooms and cook until they release their liquid and start to brown. Season with salt and pepper. Add the herbs and cook for another minute.
2. **Combine:** In a large bowl, combine sourdough bread cubes, cooked lentils, sautéed mushroom mixture, broth, and sourdough discard.
3. **Bake:** Transfer to a baking dish and bake at 350°F (175°C) for 20-25 minutes or until heated through and lightly browned.

Nutritional Values (per serving):

- Calories: 220
- Carbohydrates: 30g
- Protein: 10g
- Fat: 7g
- Sodium: 250mg
- Fiber: 6g

Cooking Tips:

- ✓ Don't overcook the lentils; they should be tender but still hold their shape.
- ✓ For a richer flavor, use a mix of dried herbs or add a splash of white wine while sautéing.

Special Diets:

- **Vegan**: Use a plant-based broth and ensure your sourdough discard is plant-based.
- **Vegetarian**: This recipe is already vegetarian-friendly!

Recipe 43: Sausage & Apple Delight

Prep Time: 20 mins | **Cook Time:** 25-30 mins | **Servings:** 6-8

Why It's Essential: This classic combination of sausage and apples delivers savory and sweet flavors with a holiday-inspired twist, enhanced by the unique tang of sourdough.

Ingredients:

- 4-5 cups cubed gluten-free sourdough bread (brown rice or sorghum starter is preferable)
- 1 pound ground breakfast sausage (mild or spicy)
- 1 cup diced apple (tart apples like Granny Smith work best)
- 1/2 cup chopped celery.
- 1/2 cup chopped onion.
- 1/4 cup chopped pecans or walnuts (optional)
- 1 tablespoon olive oil
- 1 tablespoon dried sage or poultry seasoning
- 1/2 cup vegetable broth or chicken broth
- 1/4 cup sourdough discard (any variety)
- Salt and pepper to taste

Alternative Ingredients:

- Use your favorite type of ground sausage – Italian sausage adds extra spice.
- Substitute pecans or walnuts with other nuts for additional flavor and crunch.

Step-by-Step Instructions:

1. **Cook Sausage:** In a large skillet, brown the ground sausage over medium heat, breaking it up as it cooks. Drain off any excess fat.
2. **Sauté:** Add olive oil, onion, celery, apple, and pecans (if using) to the skillet. Cook until vegetables are softened, and the apple is slightly tender-crisp. Season with salt and pepper. Add the sage or poultry seasoning.
3. **Combine:** In a large bowl, combine sourdough bread cubes, cooked sausage mixture, broth, and sourdough discard.
4. **Bake:** Transfer to a baking dish and bake at 350°F (175°C) for 25-30 minutes or until heated through and lightly browned.

Nutritional Values (per serving):

- ❖ Calories: 350
- ❖ Carbohydrates: 30g
- ❖ Protein: 20g
- ❖ Fat: 18g
- ❖ Sodium: 400mg
- ❖ Fiber: 4g

Cooking Tips:

- ✓ For a vegetarian version, use plant-based sausage crumbles and omit the nuts.
- ✓ Add a sprinkle of dried cranberries for a touch of sweetness.

Special Diets:

- This recipe is not suitable for vegetarian or vegan diets.

Recipe 44: Greek-Inspired Panzanella

Prep Time: 15 mins | **Resting Time:** 15-30 mins | **Servings:** 4-6

Why It's Essential: This salad offers a refreshing burst of Mediterranean flavors with the classic combination of tomatoes, cucumbers, olives, chickpeas, and feta, with the bright tang of red wine vinegar and sourdough.

Ingredients:

- 4-5 cups cubed gluten-free sourdough bread (crusty bread works well)
- 2 cups cherry tomatoes halved or quartered.
- 1 cup chopped cucumber.
- 1/2 cup chickpeas rinsed and drained.
- 1/4 cup chopped red onion.
- 1/4 cup crumbled feta cheese
- 3 tablespoons olive oil
- 2 tablespoons red wine vinegar
- 1 tablespoon sourdough discard (any variety)
- 1 teaspoon dried oregano
- Salt and pepper to taste

Alternative Ingredients:

- Swap cherry tomatoes for other types of tomatoes like heirloom or Roma.
- Use kalamata olives instead of chickpeas for a different flavor profile.
- Add chopped fresh herbs like parsley or mint.

Step-by-Step Instructions:

1. **Toss Bread:** In a large bowl, combine sourdough bread cubes with a drizzle of olive oil and a pinch of salt.
2. **Make Dressing:** Whisk together the remaining olive oil, red wine vinegar, sourdough discard, oregano, salt, and pepper.
3. **Combine & Rest:** Add tomatoes, cucumbers, chickpeas, onion, feta (if using), and dressing to the bowl with the bread. Toss gently and let the salad rest for 15-30 minutes to allow the bread to soak up the flavors.
4. **Serve:** Taste and adjust seasoning with salt and pepper as needed. Serve immediately.

Nutritional Values (per serving):

- Calories: 300
- Carbohydrates: 35g
- Protein: 10g
- Fat: 18g
- Sodium: 350mg
- Fiber: 6

Cooking Tips:

- Use stale bread for the best results in Panzanella.
- Add other Greek-inspired ingredients like capers, artichoke hearts, or roasted bell peppers.

Special Diets:

- **Vegetarian**: This recipe is already vegetarian-friendly!
- **Vegan**: Use a plant-based sourdough; discard and substitute the feta cheese with a vegan alternative or omit.

Chapter 11: Pretzels
(7 recipes)

Chapter 11 unfolds an inviting array of pretzel recipes, each creatively incorporating sourdough discard to infuse additional flavor and texture into this beloved snack. From the classic twists of soft pretzels to innovative stuffed bites, this section is dedicated to reimagining pretzels with a delightful sourdough twist. These seven recipes not only highlight the versatility of pretzels but also the unique tang that sourdough brings to baked goods.

Pretzels, with their distinctive chewy texture and classic knot shape, have been a favorite for generations. By adding sourdough discard to the dough, these recipes enhance the depth of flavor, bringing a new dimension to the traditional pretzel experience. Whether you're seeking a savory snack for game day, a portable treat for gatherings, or simply a delicious project for a weekend baking session, these pretzel recipes offer something for every occasion and taste preference.

In this chapter, we explore:

Recipe 45: Classic Soft Pretzels: Classic pretzel dough made with a portion of sourdough discarded for extra tang. Serve with spicy mustard!

Recipe 46: Cheesy Jalapeño Pretzel Bites: Incorporate sourdough discard into a pretzel dough, add grated cheddar cheese and diced jalapeños for a spicy kick.

Recipe 47: Cinnamon Sugar Pretzel Twists: After boiling, brush sourdough and discard pretzels with melted butter and a cinnamon-sugar mix.

Recipe 48: Ham & Cheese Stuffed Pretzels: Stuff sourdough; discard pretzel dough with diced ham and shredded cheese. Dip in a beer cheese sauce.

Recipe 49: Spiced Pumpkin Pretzel Knots: Add pumpkin puree and spices to a sourdough pretzel dough. Serve with cream cheese dip.

Recipe 50: Everything Bagel Pretzels: Incorporate sourdough, discard in the dough, then top with "everything bagel" seasoning.

Recipe 51: Herbed Garlic Pretzel Sticks: Work fresh herbs and roasted garlic into a sourdough discard pretzel dough, perfect for dipping in marinara sauce.

Each recipe includes detailed instructions on how to prepare the dough, shape the pretzels, and apply the perfect finish—whether it's a simple salt sprinkle or a more decadent topping. Tips on how to achieve the signature pretzel texture, the importance of the baking soda bath, and ideas for dips and sauces to complement your creations are also provided.

Dive into this chapter ready to twist, boil, and bake your way through a collection of recipes that celebrate the humble pretzel in all its glory, enhanced by the unique character of sourdough. Let's bring the warmth and comfort of freshly baked pretzels into your kitchen!

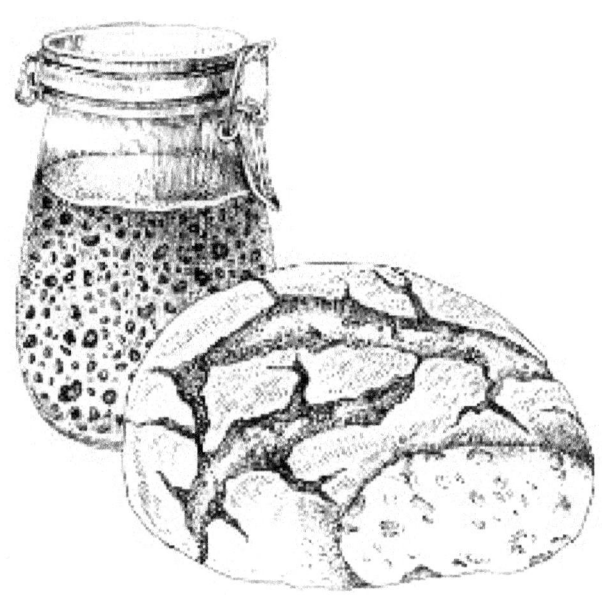

Steam Is Crucial: "Create steam in your oven during the first 20 minutes of baking by using ice cubes, a water pan, or spraying water to help the bread expand freely and form a crispy crust."

Recipe 45: Classic Soft Pretzels

Prep Time: 30 mins + Rising Time | **Cook Time:** 10-15 mins per batch | **Servings:** 8-10 pretzels

Why It's Essential: This recipe brings the classic soft pretzel experience with the added flavor dimension of sourdough. A perfect base to explore with different toppings or dips.

Ingredients:

- 1 cup warm water (100-110°F/ 38-43°C)
- 1 tablespoon sugar
- 1 teaspoon active dry yeast
- 3 1/2 cups all-purpose flour (or gluten-free blend for GF pretzels)
- 1/2 cup sourdough discard (brown rice or sorghum starter is preferable)
- 1 teaspoon salt
- 2 tablespoons melted butter.

Baking Soda Bath:

- 10 cups water
- 1/2 cup baking soda
- Coarse salt for sprinkling (optional)

Step-by-Step Instructions:

1. **Activate Yeast:** Combine warm water, sugar, and yeast in a bowl. Let stand until foamy (5-10 min).
2. **Make Dough:** In a large mixing bowl, combine flour, sourdough, discard, salt, and the activated yeast mixture. Knead until a smooth, elastic dough forms.
3. **Rise:** Place dough in a greased bowl, cover, and let rise until doubled in size (around 1-2 hours).
4. **Shape Pretzels:** Divide dough into pieces and shape into pretzels (refer to online tutorials for shaping).
5. **Baking Soda Bath:** Bring the water and baking soda to a boil in a large pot. Boil each pretzel for 30 seconds per side.
6. **Bake:** Transfer pretzels to a baking sheet lined with parchment paper. Brush with melted butter and sprinkle with coarse salt (if desired). Bake at 450°F (230°C) for 10-15 min or until golden brown.

Nutritional Values (per pretzel):

- ❖ Calories: 200
- ❖ Carbohydrates: 40g
- ❖ Protein: 6g
- ❖ Fat: 3g
- ❖ Sodium: 400mg
- ❖ Fiber: 2g

Cooking Tips:

- ✓ The baking soda bath is key for the classic pretzel flavor and color.
- ✓ Experiment with toppings! Try sesame seeds, poppy seeds, or even a cinnamon-sugar coating.

Special Diets:

- **Gluten-Free:** Use a gluten-free flour blend and ensure other ingredients are GF to make gluten-free pretzels.

Recipe 46: Cheesy Jalapeño Pretzel Bites

Prep Time: 30 mins + Rising Time | **Cook Time:** 15-20 mins | **Servings:** 20-24 pretzel bites

Why It's Essential: These pretzel bites offer a savory and satisfying flavor combo with a boost of protein from the cheese. Perfect for dipping in your favorite sauces.

Ingredients:

- Classic Soft Pretzel Dough (From Recipe #1): Follow the instructions but reserve some dough to make the bites.
- 1/2 cup shredded cheddar cheese (or a sharper variety)
- 1/4 cup finely diced jalapeño pepper (seeds removed for less heat)
- 1/4 cup finely chopped green onions (optional)
- 1 egg, beaten (for egg wash)

Alternative Ingredients:

- Use a mix of cheeses like Monterey Jack or pepper jack for extra flavor.
- Substitute jalapeño pepper with diced green bell pepper or roasted red pepper for a milder flavor.

Step-by-Step Instructions:

1. **Make Pretzel Dough:** Follow the Classic Soft Pretzel dough instructions (Recipe #1).
2. **Flavor the Bites:** Divide a portion of the dough into small pieces. Combine cheddar cheese, diced jalapeño, and green onions (optional).
3. **Stuff & Shape:** Flatten each dough piece, place a spoonful of the cheesy filling in the center, and pinch the dough to enclose the filling. Shape into bite-sized balls.
4. **Poach & Bake:** Bring a large pot of water and baking soda mixture to a boil. Poach the bites for 10-15 seconds per side. Transfer to a parchment-lined baking sheet, brush with egg wash, and bake at 425°F (220°C) for 15-20 minutes or until golden brown.

Nutritional Values (per pretzel bite):

- Calories: 80
- Carbohydrates: 10g
- Protein: 4g
- Fat: 3g
- Sodium: 150mg
- Fiber: 1g

Cooking Tips:

- ✓ Don't overstuff the bites, as the filling can leak out during baking.
- ✓ Serve with your favorite dipping sauces, like mustard, marinara sauce, or cheese sauce.

Special Diets:

- **Vegetarian**: This recipe is already vegetarian-friendly!
- **Vegan:** For a vegan version, use a vegan cheese alternative and substitute the egg wash with a plant-based alternative (like a flax egg).

Recipe 47: Cinnamon Sugar Pretzel Twists

Prep Time: 30 mins + Rising Time | **Cook Time:** 15-20 mins | **Servings:** 10-12 pretzel twists

Why It's Essential: This recipe takes the classic soft pretzel and adds a sweet cinnamon twist for a delightful treat. A perfect alternative to traditional cinnamon rolls.

Ingredients:

- Classic Soft Pretzel Dough (From Recipe #1): Follow the instructions to make the dough.
- 1/4 cup unsalted butter, melted.
- 1/2 cup granulated sugar
- 1 tablespoon ground cinnamon

Step-by-Step Instructions:

1. **Make Pretzel Dough:** Follow the Classic Soft Pretzel dough instructions (Recipe #1).
2. **Shape Twists:** Divide the dough into pieces and roll each piece into a long, thin rope. Twist the dough into a spiral shape.
3. **Poach & Brush:** Bring a large pot of water and baking soda mixture to a boil. Poach the twists for 10-15 seconds per side. Transfer to a parchment-lined baking sheet and brush with melted butter.
4. **Cinnamon Sugar Coating:** In a bowl, combine sugar and cinnamon. Sprinkle the mixture generously over the buttered twists.
5. **Bake:** Bake at 425°F (220°C) for 15-20 minutes or until golden brown.

Nutritional Values (per pretzel twist):

- Calories: 230
- Carbohydrates: 45g
- Protein: 6g
- Fat: 6g
- Sodium: 420mg
- Fiber: 2g

Cooking Tips:

- For an extra decadent treat, drizzle the twists with a simple vanilla glaze after baking.
- If you like a stronger cinnamon flavor, increase the amount of cinnamon in the sugar mixture.

Special Diets:

- **Vegan:** For a vegan version, use a vegan butter alternative.

Recipe 48: Ham & Cheese Stuffed Pretzels

Prep Time: 30 mins + Rising Time | **Cook Time:** 15-20 mins | **Servings:** 8-10 pretzels

Why It's Essential: This recipe offers a hearty and cheesy snack or meal, with the comfort food flavors of ham and cheese baked into a soft sourdough pretzel.

Ingredients:

- Classic Soft Pretzel Dough (From Recipe #1): Follow the instructions to make the dough.
- 1/2 cup diced ham.
- 1 cup shredded cheddar cheese (or your favorite melty cheese)
- 1 egg, beaten (for egg wash)

Alternative Ingredients:

- Substitute ham with other deli meats like turkey, salami, or roast beef.
- Use a variety of cheeses like Swiss, mozzarella, or provolone for a custom flavor.

Step-by-Step Instructions:

1. **Make Pretzel Dough:** Follow the Classic Soft Pretzel dough instructions (Recipe #1).
2. **Mix Filling:** In a bowl, combine diced ham and shredded cheese.
3. **Stuff & Shape:** Divide the dough into pieces. Flatten each piece, place a spoonful of the ham and cheese filling in the center, and pinch the dough to enclose the filling. Shape into small pretzel shapes.
4. **Poach & Bake:** Bring a large pot of water and baking soda mixture to a boil. Poach the pretzels for 10-15 seconds per side. Transfer to a parchment-lined baking sheet, brush with egg wash, and bake at 425°F (220°C) for 15-20 minutes or until golden brown.

Nutritional Values (per pretzel):

- Calories: 280
- Carbohydrates: 35g
- Protein: 15g
- Fat: 12g
- Sodium: 500mg
- Fiber: 2g

Cooking Tips:

- Dice the ham into small pieces so it's easy to incorporate into the pretzels.
- Serve warm with a dipping sauce like honey mustard or beer cheese sauce.

Special Diets:

- **Vegan/Vegetarian:** This recipe is not suitable for vegetarian or vegan diets.

Recipe 49: Spiced Pumpkin Pretzel Knots

Prep Time: 30 mins + Rising Time | **Cook Time:** 15-20 mins | **Servings:** 10-12 pretzel knots

Why It's Essential: This recipe brings the warm flavors of pumpkin spice into a soft and chewy pretzel, perfect for cozy autumn snacking.

Ingredients:

- Classic Soft Pretzel Dough (From Recipe #1): Modify the dough slightly by adding: * 1/2 cup pumpkin puree * 1 teaspoon pumpkin pie spice.
- For the Dipping Sauce: * 1/2 cup cream cheese, softened * 1/4 cup powdered sugar * 1 teaspoon vanilla extract * 1-2 tablespoons milk (dairy or plant-based)

Alternative Ingredients:

- Adjust the amount of pumpkin pie spice to your taste preference.

Step-by-Step Instructions:

1. **Make Pumpkin Pretzel Dough:** Follow the Classic Soft Pretzel dough instructions (Recipe #1), incorporating pumpkin puree and pumpkin pie spice into the dough.
2. **Shape Knots:** Divide the dough into pieces and roll into ropes. Shape into simple knots.
3. **Poach & Bake:** Bring a large pot of water and baking soda mixture to a boil. Poach the knots for 10-15 seconds per side. Transfer to a parchment-lined baking sheet and bake at 425°F (220°C) for 15-20 minutes or until golden brown.
4. **Make Dipping Sauce:** While the pretzels bake, whisk together cream cheese, powdered sugar, vanilla extract, and milk until smooth.
5. **Serve:** Serve pretzels warm with cream cheese dipping sauce.

Nutritional Values (per pretzel knot):

- Calories: 220
- Carbohydrates: 40g
- Protein: 5g
- Fat: 5g
- Sodium: 400mg
- Fiber: 2g

Cooking Tips:

- To shape a simple knot, take a length of dough, form a loop, and pass one end through the loop.
- Serve pretzels warm for the best texture and flavor.

Special Diets:

- **Vegetarian**: This recipe is already vegetarian-friendly!
- **Vegan:** For a vegan version, use a vegan butter alternative in the dough and a vegan cream cheese alternative for the dipping sauce.

Recipe 50: Everything Bagel Pretzels

Prep Time: 30 mins + Rising Time | **Cook Time:** 15-20 mins | **Servings:** 8-10 pretzels

Why It's Essential: This recipe brings the beloved flavor of an "everything bagel" to a soft pretzel form. Perfect for those who love a savory and crunchy snack.

Ingredients:

- Classic Soft Pretzel Dough (From Recipe #1): Follow the instructions.
- 1 egg, beaten (for egg wash)
- 2 tablespoons "Everything Bagel" seasoning (poppy seeds, sesame seeds, dried onion, garlic flakes, salt)

Step-by-Step Instructions:

1. **Make Pretzel Dough:** Follow the Classic Soft Pretzel dough instructions (Recipe #1).
2. **Shape Pretzels:** Divide the dough into pieces and shape it into your desired pretzel form (traditional twists, bites, etc.).
3. **Poach & Brush:** Bring a large pot of water and baking soda mixture to a boil. Poach the pretzels for 10-15 seconds per side. Transfer to a parchment-lined baking sheet and brush with egg wash.
4. **Add Everything Seasoning:** Sprinkle "Everything Bagel" seasoning generously over the pretzels.
5. **Bake:** Bake at 425°F (220°C) for 15-20 minutes or until golden brown.

Nutritional Values (per pretzel):

- Calories: 210
- Carbohydrates: 40g
- Protein: 6g
- Fat: 4g
- Sodium: 450mg (varies depending on "Everything Bagel" seasoning blend)
- Fiber: 2g

Cooking Tips:

- ✓ If you don't have store-bought "Everything Bagel" seasoning, make your own by combining the individual ingredients.
- ✓ Serve warm with cream cheese or other dips for an extra treat.

Special Diets:

- **Vegetarian**: This recipe is already vegetarian-friendly!
- **Vegan:** For a vegan version, substitute the egg wash with a plant-based alternative (like a flax egg).

Recipe 51: Herbed Garlic Pretzel Sticks

Prep Time: 30 mins + Rising Time | **Cook Time:** 15-20 mins | **Servings:** 10-12 pretzel sticks

Why It's Essential: This recipe offers a delicious combination of herbs and roasted garlic infused into pretzel sticks, perfect for dipping in marinara sauce or enjoying on their own.

Ingredients:

- Classic Soft Pretzel Dough (From Recipe #1): Modify the dough slightly by adding: * 2 tablespoons chopped fresh herbs (rosemary, thyme, oregano, etc.) * 2-3 cloves roasted garlic, minced.
- 1/4 cup melted butter.
- 1/4 cup grated parmesan cheese (optional)

Alternative Ingredients:

- Experiment with different herb combinations or add a pinch of red pepper flakes for a touch of spice.

Step-by-Step Instructions:

1. **Make Herbed Garlic Dough:** Follow the Classic Soft Pretzel dough instructions (Recipe #1), incorporating the chopped herbs and roasted garlic into the dough.
2. **Shape Sticks:** Divide the dough into pieces and roll it into long, thin sticks.
3. **Poach & Bake:** Bring a large pot of water and baking soda mixture to a boil. Poach the sticks for 10-15 seconds per side. Transfer to a parchment-lined baking sheet, brush with melted butter, and sprinkle with parmesan cheese (if using). Bake at 425°F (220°C) for 15-20 minutes or until golden brown.

Nutritional Values (per pretzel stick):

- Calories: 180
- Carbohydrates: 35g
- Protein: 5g
- Fat: 4g
- Sodium: 380mg
- Fiber: 2g

Cooking Tips:

- To roast garlic, cut the top off a head of garlic, drizzle with olive oil, wrap in foil, and roast at 400°F (200°C) for 30-40 minutes.
- Serve warm with your favorite dipping sauce, like marinara sauce, pesto, or even a cheesy dip.

Special Diets:

- **Vegetarian:** This recipe is already vegetarian-friendly!
- **Vegan:** For a vegan version, use a vegan butter alternative and a plant-based parmesan alternative.

Chapter 12: Beyond the Bread: Sourdough Adventures
Sourdough Pizza Crust (5 Recipes)

Chapter 12 takes us on a culinary exploration beyond traditional sourdough bread, diving into the world of sourdough pizza crusts. This chapter celebrates the versatility of sourdough, showcasing how its unique flavors and textures can transform everyday pizza into something extraordinary. Featuring five innovative pizza recipes, each utilizing a sourdough crust as the base, we invite you to expand your sourdough repertoire and bring new tastes and techniques into your home kitchen.

Sourdough pizza crusts offer a delightful twist to the classic pizza base, adding depth and tanginess that complements a variety of toppings. From exotic Mediterranean flavors to zesty Thai-inspired toppings, each recipe is designed to enhance the sourdough base and create a harmonious blend of flavors.

Whether you're a fan of meaty, veggie-packed, or uniquely topped pizzas, there's something in this chapter for everyone.

In this chapter, we explore:

Recipe 52: Mediterranean Feast Pizza: A vibrant assembly of Mediterranean favorites like pesto, feta, and olives on a millet or amaranth sourdough crust.

Recipe 53: Thai-Inspired Chicken Pizza: A fusion of Thai flavors with peanut sauce and fresh veggies on a sorghum or brown rice sourdough crust.

Recipe 54: Lentil & Veggie Lover's: A hearty, nutritious option topped with lentils and a mix of sautéed vegetables.

Recipe 55: Shrimp & Avocado Delight: A refreshing combination of shrimp, avocado, and cherry tomatoes, perfect for a light meal.

Recipe 56: Spicy Chorizo & Pineapple: A bold, spicy pizza that pairs the heat of chorizo with the sweetness of pineapple.

Each recipe includes detailed instructions on how to prepare the sourdough pizza crust, ensuring it achieves the perfect texture—crispy on the outside, soft and chewy on the inside. We'll also provide tips for juggling fermentation times and baking techniques to get the best results from your sourdough crust.
Embark on these sourdough adventures to discover how simple it is to incorporate global flavors into your homemade pizzas. This chapter is not just about creating meals; it's about experiencing the joy of baking and the endless possibilities that sourdough brings to the table. Get ready to roll out your dough, top it creatively, and bake up a storm as you master the art of sourdough pizza making.

Recipe 52: Mediterranean Feast Pizza

Prep Time: 20 mins (+ dough rising time) | **Cook Time**: 15-20 mins

Ingredients:

Sourdough Pizza Dough:

- 1 cup sourdough discard (millet or amaranth starter preferred)
- 1 1/4 cups warm water
- 1 teaspoon sugar or honey
- 1 tablespoon olive oil
- 1 teaspoon salt
- 3-3 1/2 cups all-purpose flour

Toppings:

- 1/2 cup pesto
- 1/2 cup crumbled feta cheese
- 1/2 cup roasted red peppers (jarred or homemade)
- 1/4 cup artichoke hearts, sliced.
- 1/4 cup kalamata olives, sliced.
- 1/2 cup fresh spinach

Best Sourdough Starter:

- ✓ A millet or amaranth starter adds a subtle nutty complexity that complements the Mediterranean toppings.

Step-by-Step Instructions:

1. Make Sourdough Pizza Dough: Follow your favorite sourdough pizza dough recipe using the listed ingredients. A basic process typically involves activating the starter with water and sugar/honey, adding olive oil and salt, then gradually incorporating flour until a smooth dough forms. Let the dough rise according to the recipe instructions.
2. Prep Toppings: While dough rises, slice roasted red peppers, artichoke hearts, and olives, if necessary.
3. Assemble Pizza: Preheat oven to 450°F (230°C). Stretch or roll out the dough on a lightly floured surface or pizza stone. Spread pesto evenly over the dough. Top with feta cheese, roasted red peppers, artichoke hearts, olives, and spinach.
4. Bake: Bake for 15-20 minutes, or until the crust is golden brown and the cheese is melted and bubbly.

Nutritional Values (per slice - based on an 8-slice pizza):

- ❖ Calories: 350
- ❖ Carbohydrates: 45g
- ❖ Protein: 15g
- ❖ Fat: 15g
- ❖ Sodium: 600mg
- ❖ Fiber: 4g

Cooking Tips:

- ✓ If you don't have pesto, you can use a thin layer of marinara sauce.
- ✓ Add a sprinkle of dried oregano or thyme for extra flavor.

Recipe 53: Thai-Inspired Chicken Pizza

Prep Time: 20 mins (+ dough rising time) | **Cook Time:** 15-20 mins

Ingredients:

Sourdough Pizza Dough:

- 1 cup sourdough discard (brown rice or sorghum starter preferred)
- 1 1/4 cups warm water
- 1 teaspoon sugar or honey
- 1 tablespoon olive oil
- 1 teaspoon salt
- 3-3 1/2 cups all-purpose flour

Toppings:

- 1/2 cup peanut sauce
- 1 cup cooked shredded chicken.
- 1/2 cup shredded carrots
- 1/4 cup bean sprouts
- 1/4 cup chopped peanuts.
- 1/4 cup fresh cilantro, chopped.

Alternative Ingredients:

- ✓ Substitute chicken with tofu or shrimp for a different protein source.
- ✓ If you don't have peanut sauce, use a combination of peanut butter, soy sauce, lime juice, and a touch of brown sugar.

Step-by-Step Instructions:

1. **Make Sourdough Pizza Dough:** (Follow the same preparation as in Recipe #1)
2. **Prep Toppings:** While the dough rises, cook and shred the chicken, shred the carrots, and chop the peanuts and cilantro.
3. **Assemble Pizza:** Preheat oven to 450°F (230°C). Stretch or roll out the dough on a lightly floured surface or pizza stone. Spread peanut sauce evenly over the dough. Top with shredded chicken, carrots, bean sprouts, peanuts, and fresh cilantro.
4. **Bake:** Bake for 15-20 minutes, or until the crust is golden brown and the toppings are heated through.

Serving Suggestions:

- ✓ Drizzle with a little sriracha sauce for an extra kick of heat.
- ✓ Serve with a side of Asian-inspired slaw for a complete meal.

Nutritional Values (per slice - based on an 8-slice pizza):

- ❖ Calories: 380
- ❖ Carbohydrates: 40g
- ❖ Protein: 25g
- ❖ Fat: 18g
- ❖ Sodium: 550mg
- ❖ Fiber: 4g

Cooking Tips:

- ✓ Use pre-cooked or rotisserie chicken for convenience.
- ✓ Add a sprinkle of sesame seeds on the crust before baking for extra flavor.

Recipe 54: Lentil & Veggie Lover's Pizza

Prep Time: 20 mins (+ dough rising time) | **Cook Time:** 15-20 mins

Ingredients:

Sourdough Pizza Dough:

- 1 cup sourdough discard (any starter will work)
- 1 1/4 cups warm water
- 1 teaspoon sugar or honey
- 1 tablespoon olive oil
- 1 teaspoon salt
- 3-3 1/2 cups all-purpose flour

Toppings:

- 1/2 cup marinara sauce
- 1 cup cooked lentils
- 1/2 cup sautéed mushrooms
- 1/4 cup sliced onions.
- 1/4 cup chopped bell peppers (any color)
- 1/4 cup nutritional yeast

Alternative Ingredients:

- ✓ Substitute lentils with cooked beans (black beans, chickpeas, etc.)
- ✓ Use your favorite combination of vegetables.

Step-by-Step Instructions:

1. **Make Sourdough Pizza Dough:** (Follow the same preparation as in Recipe #1)
2. **Sauté Veggies:** While dough rises, sauté onions and mushrooms in a bit of olive oil until softened. Add chopped bell peppers and cook for a minute more.
3. **Assemble Pizza:** Preheat oven to 450°F (230°C). Stretch or roll out the dough on a lightly floured surface or pizza stone. Spread marinara sauce evenly over the dough. Top with cooked lentils, sautéed vegetables, and a sprinkle of nutritional yeast.
4. **Bake:** Bake for 15-20 minutes, or until the crust is golden brown and the toppings are heated through.

Serving Suggestions:

- Serve with a side salad for a complete and balanced meal.

Nutritional Values (per slice - based on an 8-slice pizza):

- ❖ Calories: 300
- ❖ Carbohydrates: 40g
- ❖ Protein: 15g
- ❖ Fat: 10g
- ❖ Sodium: 400mg
- ❖ Fiber: 8g

Cooking Tips:

- ✓ Add a sprinkle of red pepper flakes for a touch of heat.
- ✓ Top with a drizzle of balsamic glaze after baking for an extra layer of flavor.

Recipe 55: Shrimp & Avocado Delight

Prep Time: 20 mins (+ dough rising time) | **Cook Time:** 15-20 mins

Ingredients:

Sourdough Pizza Dough:

- 1 cup sourdough discard (any starter will work)
- 1 1/4 cups warm water
- 1 teaspoon sugar or honey
- 1 tablespoon olive oil
- 1 teaspoon salt
- 3-3 1/2 cups all-purpose flour

Toppings:

- 1/4 cup olive oil
- 2 cloves garlic, minced.
- 1/2-pound medium shrimp, peeled and deveined
- 1/4 teaspoon salt
- 1/4 teaspoon black pepper
- 1/4 cup lemon juice
- 1/2 cup cherry or grape tomatoes, halved.
- 1 avocado, sliced.
- 1/4 cup fresh basil, chopped.

Alternative Ingredients:

- ✓ Substitute shrimp with cooked scallops or flaked white fish.
- ✓ Use your favorite type of tomatoes.

Step-by-Step Instructions:

1. **Make Sourdough Pizza Dough:** (Follow the same preparation as in Recipe #1)
2. **Cook Shrimp:** While the dough rises, heat olive oil in a skillet. Add garlic and cook for 30 seconds. Add shrimp, salt, and pepper. Cook until shrimp turn pink and are cooked through. Remove the shrimp from the skillet.
3. **Assemble Pizza:** Preheat oven to 450°F (230°C). Stretch or roll out the dough on a lightly floured surface or pizza stone. Drizzle with a bit of garlicky olive oil from the pan. Top with cooked shrimp, tomatoes, avocado slices, and a sprinkle of fresh basil.
4. **Bake:** Bake for 15-20 minutes, or until the crust is golden brown and the toppings are heated through.

Nutritional Values (per slice - based on an 8-slice pizza):

- ❖ Calories: 320
- ❖ Carbohydrates: 35g
- ❖ Protein: 20g
- ❖ Fat: 15g
- ❖ Sodium: 450mg
- ❖ Fiber: 4g

Cooking Tips:

- ✓ Don't overcrowd the pizza with toppings to ensure even cooking.
- ✓ Add avocado slices just before serving to maintain their freshness.

Special Diets:

- **Gluten-Free:** For a gluten-free version, use a gluten-free pizza dough recipe.

Recipe 56: Spicy Chorizo & Pineapple

Prep Time: 20 mins (+ dough rising time) | **Cook Time:** 15-20 mins

Ingredients:

Sourdough Pizza Dough:

- 1 cup sourdough discard (any starter will work)
- 1 1/4 cups warm water
- 1 teaspoon sugar or honey
- 1 tablespoon olive oil
- 1 teaspoon salt
- 3-3 1/2 cups all-purpose flour

Toppings:

- 1/2 cup chipotle-infused tomato sauce (or regular tomato sauce + chipotle powder)
- 1/2 cup crumbled chorizo
- 1/2 cup diced pineapple.
- 1/4 cup sliced red onion.
- 1/4 cup chopped fresh cilantro.

Alternative Ingredients:

- ✓ Substitute chorizo with spicy Italian sausage.
- ✓ Add sliced jalapeños for an extra kick of heat.

Step-by-Step Instructions:

1. Make Sourdough Pizza Dough: (Follow the same preparation as in Recipe #1)
2. **Cook Chorizo:** While the dough rises, cook crumbled chorizo in a skillet over medium heat until browned and cooked through.
3. **Assemble Pizza:** Preheat oven to 450°F (230°C). Stretch or roll out the dough on a lightly floured surface or pizza stone. Spread chipotle-infused tomato sauce evenly over the dough. Top with chorizo, pineapple, red onion, and a sprinkle of cilantro.
4. **Bake:** Bake for 15-20 minutes, or until the crust is golden brown and the toppings are heated through.

Nutritional Values (per slice - based on an 8-slice pizza):

- ❖ Calories: 350
- ❖ Carbohydrates: 35g
- ❖ Protein: 18g
- ❖ Fat: 18g
- ❖ Sodium: 550mg
- ❖ Fiber: 3g

Cooking Tips:

- ✓ If you don't have chipotle-infused sauce, add a pinch of chipotle powder to regular tomato sauce.
- ✓ Use fresh pineapple for the best flavor.

Special Diets:

- **Gluten-Free:** For a gluten-free version, Use a gluten-free pizza dough recipe.

Chapter 13: Sourdough Bagels (5 Recipes)

Welcome to "Sourdough Bagels," a chapter that invites you to explore the delightful versatility of sourdough through the art of bagel making. Here, the classic bagel is reimagined with the unique tang and texture of sourdough, creating a series of recipes that infuse traditional techniques with innovative, flavorful twists. Each recipe in this chapter utilizes sourdough discard, ensuring that no part of your sourdough starter goes to waste while bringing an extra depth of flavor to these beloved bread rings.

Sourdough bagels offer a fantastic way to experiment with different flavors and ingredients, turning the ordinary bagel experience into something extraordinary. From protein-packed creations to sweet and savory delights, these bagels are perfect for any meal, providing satisfying textures and robust flavors that are sure to impress.

Explore the Art of Sourdough Bagels:

- **Recipe 57: Protein Power Bagel** Boost your morning with a bagel that not only tastes great but also fuels your day. This protein-rich bagel features protein powder, ground flaxseeds, and a sorghum-based starter. It is perfect for a post-workout meal or a hearty breakfast topped with cream cheese and smoked salmon.

- **Recipe 58: Spiced Lentil & Quinoa Bagel** Dive into the earthy flavors of red lentils and quinoa, mixed into sourdough bagel dough with a touch of cumin and coriander for a fragrant and nutritious option. The amaranth starter enhances the natural nuttiness of the grains, creating a bagel that's both hearty and flavorful.

- **Recipe 59: "Everything" Meets Sourdough** Combine the iconic taste of an "everything bagel" with the distinctive tang of sourdough. This recipe melds poppy seeds, sesame seeds, onion flakes, and garlic powder with sourdough discard, offering a bagel that's robust in flavor and perfect for any cream cheese schmear.

- **Recipe 60: Blueberry Almond Swirl Bagel** Sweet meets sourdough in this delightful bagel featuring chopped almonds and dried blueberries. The use of a brown rice starter provides a neutral base that allows the sweetness of the berries and the nuttiness of the almonds to shine, complemented by a dollop of honey-sweetened cream cheese.

- **Recipe 61: Sundried Tomato & Olive Bagel** For a taste of the Mediterranean, this bagel incorporates sundried tomatoes and chopped kalamata olives into the dough, creating a savory treat that pairs wonderfully with a variety of toppings or enjoys simply on its own.

Perfecting Your Sourdough Bagel Technique

Beyond recipes, this chapter provides essential tips for working with sourdough in bagel dough, from maintaining perfect hydration to achieving the ideal chewiness. You'll learn how to boil and bake sourdough bagels to perfection, ensuring they have the classic shiny crust and tender crumb that make bagels so beloved.

Step into "Sourdough Bagels" to expand your baking repertoire and discover new ways to enjoy sourdough. Whether you're a seasoned baker or new to the world of sourdough, these bagels are sure to add a delicious twist to your culinary creations, making every breakfast, lunch, or snack time a delightful experience.

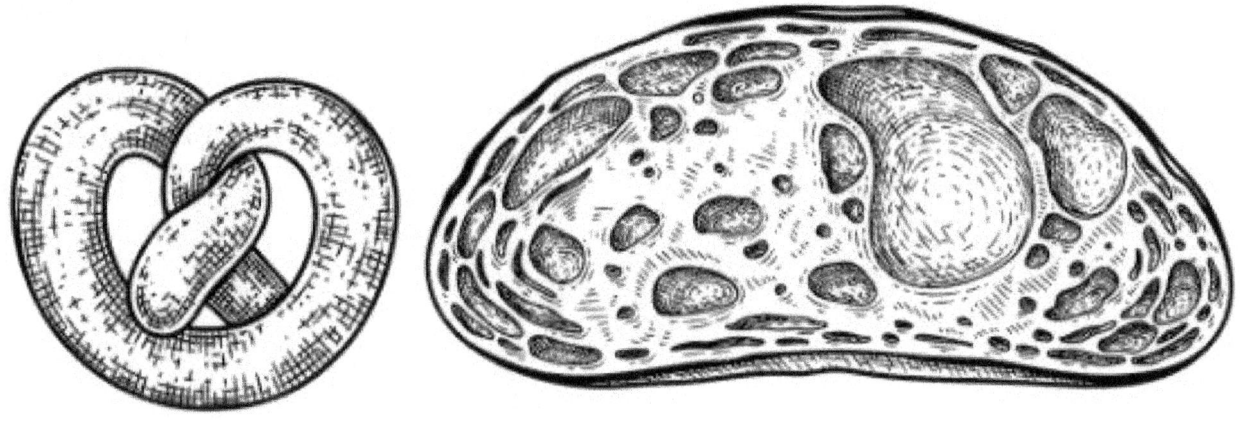

Cool Completely Before Slicing: "Allow your sourdough bread to cool completely on a wire rack before slicing to prevent a gummy texture and fully develop the flavors."

Recipe 57: Protein Power Bagel

Prep Time: 30 mins (+ dough rising time) | **Cook Time:** 20-25 mins

Ingredients:

Sourdough Bagel Dough:

- 1 cup sourdough discard (brown rice or sorghum starter works best)
- 1 1/4 cups warm water
- 1 tablespoon honey or maple syrup
- 1 tablespoon olive oil
- 1 teaspoon salt
- 1/4 cup protein powder (vanilla or unflavored)
- 1/4 cup ground flaxseeds
- 3-3 1/2 cups all-purpose flour

Toppings:

- Smoked salmon
- Cream cheese!
- Capers (optional)
    Thinly sliced red onion (optional)

Step-by-Step Instructions:

1. **Make Sourdough Bagel Dough:** Follow a basic sourdough bagel dough recipe. Combine all dough ingredients, kneading until a smooth dough forms. Let it rise according to recipe instructions.
2. **Shape & Boil:** After the dough rises, divide it into equal portions, shape it into bagels, and let them rest. Boil the bagels in a large pot of water with a touch of baking soda (for the classic chewy texture).
3. **Bake:** After boiling, transfer the bagels to a baking sheet lined with parchment paper. Bake in a preheated oven at 425°F (220°C) for 20-25 minutes or until golden brown.
4. **Assemble:** Serve the bagels sliced, topped with cream cheese, smoked salmon, capers (if desired), and thinly sliced red onion.

Nutritional Values (per bagel):

- ❖ Calories: 400
- ❖ Carbohydrates: 50g
- ❖ Protein: 25g
- ❖ Fat: 15g
- ❖ Sodium: 500mg
- ❖ Fiber: 6

Cooking Tips:

- ✓ Please choose your favorite protein powder flavor, keeping in mind how it will pair with your toppings.
- ✓ If you don't have smoked salmon, substitute it with other thinly sliced smoked fish.

Special Diets:

- **Gluten-Free:** For a gluten-free version, use a gluten-free bagel dough recipe.

Best Sourdough Starter:

> Sorghum or brown rice starter provides a neutral flavor base that lets the protein powder and flaxseeds shine.

Recipe 58: Spiced Lentil & Quinoa

Prep Time: 30 mins (+ dough rising time + lentil and quinoa cooking) | **Cook Time:** 20-25 mins.

Ingredients:

Sourdough Bagel Dough:

- 1 cup sourdough discard (amaranth starter preferred)
- 1 1/4 cups warm water
- 1 tablespoon honey or maple syrup
- 1 tablespoon olive oil
- 1 teaspoon salt
- 1/2 cup cooked red lentils.
- 1/4 cup cooked quinoa
- 1 teaspoon cumin powder
- 1/2 teaspoon coriander powder
- 3-3 1/2 cups all-purpose flour

Alternative Ingredients:

Substitute red lentils with cooked green or brown lentils.

If you don't have quinoa, add some extra lentils for added protein.

Step-by-Step Instructions:

1. **Make Sourdough Bagel Dough:** Follow a basic sourdough bagel dough recipe. Combine all dough ingredients, including the cooked lentils, quinoa, and spices. Knead until a smooth dough forms. Let it rise according to recipe instructions.
2. **Shape & Boil:** After the dough rises, divide it into equal portions, shape it into bagels, and let them rest. Boil the bagels in a large pot of water with a touch of baking soda (for the classic chewy texture).
3. **Bake:** After boiling, transfer the bagels to a baking sheet lined with parchment paper. Bake in a preheated oven at 425°F (220°C) for 20-25 minutes or until golden brown.

Nutritional Values (per bagel):

- Calories: 320
- Carbohydrates: 55g
- Protein: 15g
- Fat: 8g
- Sodium: 450mg
- Fiber: 8g

Cooking Tips:

- Make sure your lentils and quinoa are well-cooked before adding them to the dough.
- Add a pinch of turmeric to the dough for a vibrant yellow color.

Special Diets:

- **Vegan**: This recipe is already vegan-friendly! For a gluten-free version, use a gluten-free bagel dough recipe.

Recipe 59: "Everything" Meets Sourdough

Prep Time: 30 mins (+ dough rising time) | **Cook Time:** 20-25 mins

Ingredients:

Sourdough Bagel Dough:

- 1 cup sourdough discard (any starter will work)
- 1 1/4 cups warm water
- 1 tablespoon honey or maple syrup
- 1 tablespoon olive oil
- 1 teaspoon salt
- 3-3 1/2 cups all-purpose flour

"Everything" Topping:

- 1 tablespoon poppy seeds
- 1 tablespoon sesame seeds
- 1 teaspoon dried onion flakes
- 1 teaspoon dried garlic powder
- 1/2 teaspoon coarse salt

Step-by-Step Instructions:

1. **Make Sourdough Bagel Dough:** Follow a basic sourdough bagel dough recipe. Combine all dough ingredients, kneading until a smooth dough forms. Let it rise according to recipe instructions.
2. **Make Topping:** In a small bowl, combine the poppy seeds, sesame seeds, onion flakes, garlic powder, and coarse salt.
3. **Shape & Boil:** After the dough rises, divide it into equal portions, shape it into bagels, and let them rest. Boil the bagels in a large pot of water with a touch of baking soda (for the classic chewy texture).
4. **Add Topping & Bake:** After boiling, brush the bagels with a beaten egg (or water for an egg-free version) and sprinkle generously with the "everything" seasoning mix. Bake in a preheated oven at 425°F (220°C) for 20-25 minutes or until golden brown.

Nutritional Values (per bagel):

- Calories: 350
- Carbohydrates: 55g
- Protein: 12g
- Fat: 12g
- Sodium: 550mg
- Fiber: 4g

Cooking Tips:

- Toast your bagels before serving for extra crunch.
- Store leftover bagels in an airtight container at room temperature for a day or two.

Special Diets:

- **Vegan:** For a vegan version, use an egg wash substitute, such as water or a flax egg.
- **Gluten-Free:** For a gluten-free version, use a gluten-free bagel dough recipe.

Recipe 60: Blueberry Almond Swirl

Prep Time: 30 mins (+ dough rising time) | **Cook Time:** 20-25 mins

Ingredients:

Sourdough Bagel Dough:

- 1 cup sourdough discard (brown rice starter preferred)
- 1 1/4 cups warm water
- 1 tablespoon honey or maple syrup
- 1 tablespoon olive oil
- 1 teaspoon salt
- 3-3 1/2 cups all-purpose flour

Filling:

- 1/2 cup dried blueberries
- 1/4 cup chopped almonds.
- 2 tablespoons brown sugar
- 1 teaspoon ground cinnamon

Alternative Ingredients:

- Substitute dried blueberries with fresh blueberries (slightly mashed) or other dried fruits like cranberries or raisins.
- Use other nuts like pecans or walnuts instead of almonds.

Step-by-Step Instructions:

1. **Make Sourdough Bagel Dough:** Follow a basic sourdough bagel recipe. Combine all dough ingredients, kneading until a smooth dough forms. Let it rise according to recipe instructions.
2. **Make Filling:** In a bowl, combine dried blueberries, chopped almonds, brown sugar, and cinnamon.
3. **Shape & Fill:** After the dough rises, divide it into equal portions. Roll out each portion into a rectangle. Spread a thin layer of the blueberry-almond filling onto each rectangle. Roll up the dough tightly, sealing the edges. Shape into bagels and let rest.
4. **Boil & Bake:** Boil the bagels in a large pot of water with a touch of baking soda (for the classic chewy texture). After boiling, transfer the bagels to a baking sheet lined with parchment paper. Bake in a preheated oven at 425°F (220°C) for 20-25 minutes or until golden brown.

Serving Suggestions:

- ✓ Serve warm with honey-sweetened cream cheese for a delightful breakfast or snack.

Nutritional Values (per bagel):

- ❖ Calories: 380
- ❖ Carbohydrates: 60g
- ❖ Protein: 12g
- ❖ Fat: 13g
- ❖ Sodium: 450mg
- ❖ Fiber: 5

Cooking Tips:

- ✓ To check if the dough has risen enough, try the 'poke test': gently poke the dough with your finger. If the indentation springs back slowly, it's ready.
- ✓ Don't overfill the bagels, as the filling can expand during baking and make shaping difficult.

Recipe 61: Sundried Tomato & Olive

Prep Time: 30 mins (+ dough rising time) | **Cook Time:** 20-25 mins

Ingredients:

Sourdough Bagel Dough:

- 1 cup sourdough discard (any starter will work)
- 1 1/4 cups warm water
- 1 tablespoon honey or maple syrup
- 1 tablespoon olive oil
- 1 teaspoon salt
- 3-3 1/2 cups all-purpose flour

Filling:

- 1/4 cup chopped sundried tomatoes (packed in oil)
- 1/4 cup chopped kalamata olives.
- 1 teaspoon dried oregano

Alternative Ingredients:

- Substitute kalamata olives with other types of olives, like green olives or black olives.
- Add a sprinkle of dried basil or rosemary for additional herbal notes.

Step-by-Step Instructions:

1. **Make Sourdough Bagel Dough:** Follow a basic sourdough bagel dough recipe. Combine all dough ingredients, kneading until a smooth dough forms. Let it rise according to recipe instructions.
2. **Incorporate Filling:** After the dough rises, gently knead in the chopped sundried tomatoes, chopped olives, and dried oregano.
3. **Shape & Boil:** Divide the dough into equal portions, shape it into bagels, and let them rest. Boil the bagels in a large pot of water with a touch of baking soda (for the classic chewy texture).
4. **Bake:** After boiling, transfer the bagels to a baking sheet lined with parchment paper. Bake in a preheated oven at 425°F (220°C) for 20-25 minutes or until golden brown.

Serving Suggestions:

- ✓ Enjoy warm with a spread of cream cheese or whipped ricotta, and top with fresh herbs like basil or chives.

Nutritional Values (per bagel):

- ❖ Calories: 350
- ❖ Carbohydrates: 55g
- ❖ Protein: 12g
- ❖ Fat: 13g
- ❖ Sodium: 600mg
- ❖ Fiber: 4g

Cooking Tips:

- ✓ Drain the sundried tomatoes of excess oil before adding them to the dough.
- ✓ If you like a more intense olive flavor, use more olives in the filling.

Chapter 14: Sourdough Cinnamon Rolls (5 Recipes)

Welcome to "Sourdough Cinnamon Rolls," a chapter that transforms the classic cinnamon roll into an extraordinary adventure with the unique twist of sourdough. This chapter delves into the delightful world of cinnamon rolls, infusing them with the complexity and depth of sourdough discard to enhance both flavor and texture. Each recipe is carefully crafted to bring out the best in traditional flavors while introducing exciting new combinations, ensuring that every roll is a discovery of its own.

Sourdough discard not only adds a tangy counterpoint to the sweet richness of cinnamon rolls but also improves the texture, making them lighter and more flavorful. These recipes explore various fillings and toppings that complement the distinctive taste of sourdough, from fruits and nuts to spices and chocolates, offering a cinnamon roll for every occasion and taste preference.

Discover the Rolls of Your Dreams:

- **Recipe 62: High-Protein Cinnamon Rolls** Perfect for fitness enthusiasts, these cinnamon rolls are boosted with protein powder and baked using a sourdough discard base. The rolls are then topped with a protein-rich cream cheese frosting, making them a guilt-free indulgence that fuels your day.

- **Recipe 63: Pumpkin Spice Swirl** Embrace the essence of fall with pumpkin puree and a medley of spices mixed into the dough, swirled with classic cinnamon sugar. These rolls are a warm, comforting treat that perfectly captures the season's flavors.

- **Recipe 64: Apple Walnut Delight** Incorporate the crispness of apples and the crunch of walnuts into your rolls, creating a delightful texture contrast. The amaranth starter adds a beautiful earthiness, complemented by a sweet drizzle of caramel sauce.

- **Recipe 65: Tropical Twist** Bring a bit of the tropics to your kitchen with cinnamon rolls filled with pineapple, coconut, and brown sugar. The tropical fruits provide a fresh burst of flavor, enhanced by a glaze subtly flavored with rum extract.

- **Recipe 66: Chocolate & Cherry Indulgence** For chocolate lovers, these cinnamon rolls are a dream. The dough is spread with a rich chocolate hazelnut paste and sprinkled with dried cherries before rolling. Each bite is a decadent, gooey delight that's both satisfying and luxurious.

Elevate Your Baking Skills

This chapter goes beyond recipes to offer tips on working with sourdough discard in sweet doughs, ensuring your cinnamon rolls are always fluffy and flavorful. You'll learn the nuances of fermenting and proofing times to get the best results from your sourdough cinnamon rolls, turning them into not just a treat but a centerpiece for breakfasts, brunches, or desserts.

Dive into "Sourdough Cinnamon Rolls" and let these recipes inspire you to bake with passion and creativity. Whether you're hosting a special brunch or simply treating yourself, these cinnamon rolls promise to elevate your baking repertoire and impress your taste buds with every spiral of sweet, tangy dough.

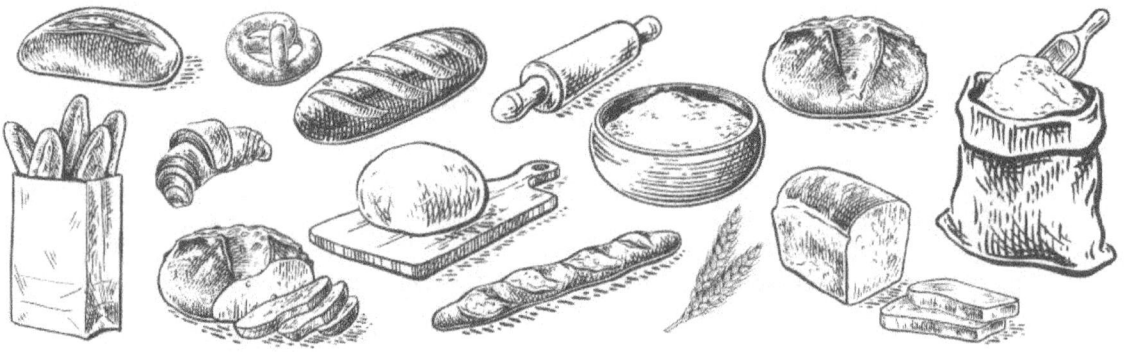

Recipe 62: High-Protein Cinnamon Rolls

Prep Time: 30 mins (+ dough rising time) | **Cook Time:** 25-30 mins

Ingredients:

Sourdough Cinnamon Roll Dough:

- 1 cup sourdough discard (brown rice or sorghum starter preferred)
- 1/2 cup warm water
- 1/4 cup unsweetened almond milk (or other low-carb milk)
- 1 large egg
- 1 tablespoon melted coconut oil or butter.
- 1/4 cup protein powder (vanilla or unflavored)
- 1/4 cup granulated sweetener of choice (monk fruit, stevia, etc.)
- 1 teaspoon vanilla extract
- 1 teaspoon baking powder
- 1/2 teaspoon salt
- 2-2 1/2 cups all-purpose flour

Filling:

- 2 tablespoons melted coconut oil or butter.
- 1/4 cup granulated sweetener of choice (monk fruit, stevia, etc.)
- 1 tablespoon ground cinnamon

Protein Frosting:

- 1/2 cup cream cheese, softened.
- 1/4 cup protein powder (vanilla or unflavored)
- 2-3 tablespoons unsweetened almond milk (or other low-carb milk)
- 1 teaspoon vanilla extract

Step-by-Step Instructions:

1. **Make Sourdough Dough:** Combine sourdough discard, water, almond milk, egg, melted coconut oil, protein powder, sweetener, vanilla, baking powder, and salt. Gradually add flour until the dough forms. Knead until smooth and elastic. Let rise in a warm place until doubled in size.
2. **Make Filling:** In a small bowl, combine melted coconut oil or butter, sweetener, and cinnamon.
3. **Roll & Fill:** Roll out the dough into a rectangle. Spread filling evenly. Roll up tightly, seal the edge, and cut into rolls. Place in a greased baking dish. Let rise again until slightly puffy.
4. **Bake:** Bake in a preheated oven at 375°F (190°C) for 25-30 minutes or until golden brown.
5. **Make Frosting:** While the rolls bake, beat together cream cheese, protein powder, almond milk, and vanilla until smooth. Spread on slightly cooled rolls.

Nutritional Values (per roll):

- Calories: 250
- Carbohydrates: 25g
- Protein: 15g
- Fat: 13g
- Sodium: 250mg
- Fiber: 3g

Cooking Tips:

- ✓ Choose your preferred protein powder flavor to complement the cinnamon rolls.
- ✓ If you don't have protein powder, use an additional 1/4 cup of flour in the dough.

Recipe 63: Pumpkin Spice Swirl

Prep Time: 30 mins (+ dough rising time) | **Cook Time:** 25-30 mins

Ingredients:

Sourdough Cinnamon Roll Dough:

- 1 cup sourdough discard (any starter will work)
- 1/2 cup warm water
- 1/4 cup unsweetened almond milk (or other low-carb milk)
- 1/4 cup pumpkin puree
- 1 tablespoon melted coconut oil or butter.
- 1/4 cup granulated sweetener of choice (monk fruit, stevia, etc.)
- 1 teaspoon pumpkin pie spice
- 1/2 teaspoon ground cinnamon
- 1 teaspoon vanilla extract
- 1 teaspoon baking powder
- 1/2 teaspoon salt
- 2-2 1/2 cups all-purpose flour

Filling:

- 2 tablespoons melted coconut oil or butter.
- 1/4 cup granulated sweetener of choice (monk fruit, stevia, etc.)
- 1 tablespoon ground cinnamon

Alternative Ingredients

- Substitute pumpkin puree with mashed sweet potato for a similar flavor and texture.
- If you don't have pumpkin pie spice, make your own blend using cinnamon, nutmeg, ginger, and cloves.

Step-by-Step Instructions:

1. **Make Sourdough Dough:** Combine sourdough discard, water, almond milk, pumpkin puree, melted coconut oil, sweetener, pumpkin pie spice, cinnamon, vanilla, baking powder, and salt. Gradually add flour until the dough forms. Knead until smooth and elastic. Let rise in a warm place until doubled in size.
2. **Make Filling:** In a small bowl, combine melted coconut oil or butter, sweetener, and cinnamon.
3. **Roll & Fill:** Roll out the dough into a rectangle. Spread filling evenly. Roll up tightly, seal the edge, and cut into rolls. Place in a greased baking dish. Let rise again until slightly puffy.
4. **Bake:** Bake in a preheated oven at 375°F (190°C) for 25-30 minutes or until golden brown.

Nutritional Values (per roll):

- Calories: 220
- Carbohydrates: 30g
- Protein: 5g
- Fat: 10g
- Sodium: 200mg
- Fiber: 4g

Cooking Tips:

- ✓ For a more intense pumpkin flavor, add a tablespoon or two of molasses to the dough.
- ✓ Experiment with other warm spices like ginger or cardamom in the filling.

Recipe 64: Apple Walnut Delight

Prep Time: 30 mins (+ dough rising time) | **Cook Time:** 25-30 mins

Ingredients:

Sourdough Cinnamon Roll Dough:

- 1 cup sourdough discard (amaranth starter preferred)
- 1/2 cup warm water
- 1/4 cup unsweetened almond milk (or other low-carb milk)
- 1 large egg
- 1 tablespoon melted coconut oil or butter.
- 1/4 cup granulated sweetener of choice (monk fruit, stevia, etc.)
- 1 teaspoon ground cinnamon
- 1/2 teaspoon vanilla extract
- 1 teaspoon baking powder
- 1/2 teaspoon salt
- 2-2 1/2 cups all-purpose flour

Filling:

- 1/2 cup finely diced apple.
- 1/4 cup chopped walnuts.
- 2 tablespoons melted coconut oil or butter.
- 1/4 cup granulated sweetener of choice (monk fruit, stevia, etc.)
- 1 teaspoon ground cinnamon

Optional Caramel Drizzle:

- 1/4 cup sugar-free caramel sauce

Alternative Ingredients

- Use other types of nuts, like pecans or almonds, in place of walnuts.
- Substitute the apple with pear or other seasonal fruit.

Step-by-Step Instructions:

1. **Make Sourdough Dough:** Combine sourdough discard, water, almond milk, egg, melted coconut oil, sweetener, cinnamon, vanilla, baking powder, and salt. Gradually add flour until the dough forms. Knead until smooth and elastic. Let rise in a warm place until doubled in size.
2. **Make Filling:** In a small bowl, combine diced apple, walnuts melted coconut oil or butter, sweetener, and cinnamon.
3. **Roll & Fill:** Roll out the dough into a rectangle. Spread filling evenly. Roll up tightly, seal the edge, and cut into rolls. Place in a greased baking dish. Let rise again until slightly puffy.
4. **Bake:** Bake in a preheated oven at 375°F (190°C) for 25-30 minutes or until golden brown.
5. **Caramel Drizzle:** If desired, warm up sugar-free caramel sauce and drizzle over the slightly cooled rolls.

Nutritional Values (per roll):

- Calories: 250
- Carbohydrates: 30g
- Protein: 6g
- Fat: 13g
- Sodium: 220mg
- Fiber: 4g

Cooking Tips:

- Finely dice the apples for easier rolling and even distribution.
- Toast the walnuts before adding to the filling for an extra layer of flavor.

Recipe 65: Tropical Twist

Prep Time: 30 mins (+ dough rising time) | Cook Time: 25-30 mins

Ingredients:

Sourdough Cinnamon Roll Dough:

- 1 cup sourdough discard (any starter will work)
- 1/2 cup warm water
- 1/4 cup unsweetened almond milk (or other low-carb milk)
- 1 large egg
- 1 tablespoon melted coconut oil or butter.
- 1/4 cup granulated sweetener of choice (monk fruit, stevia, etc.)
- 1/2 teaspoon vanilla extract
- 1 teaspoon baking powder
- 1/2 teaspoon salt
- 2-2 1/2 cups all-purpose flour

Filling:

- 1/2 cup diced pineapple (fresh or canned, well-drained)
- 1/4 cup shredded coconut
- 2 tablespoons brown sugar
- 1/2 teaspoon rum extract (or vanilla extract)

Alternative Ingredients:

- Use other tropical fruits like mango or papaya in place of pineapple.

Step-by-Step Instructions:

1. **Make Sourdough Dough:** Combine sourdough discard, water, almond milk, egg, melted coconut oil, sweetener, vanilla, baking powder, and salt. Gradually add flour until the dough forms. Knead until smooth and elastic. Let rise in a warm place until doubled in size.
2. **Make Filling:** In a small bowl, combine diced pineapple, shredded coconut, brown sugar, and rum extract.
3. **Roll & Fill:** Roll out the dough into a rectangle. Spread filling evenly. Roll up tightly, seal the edge, and cut into rolls. Place in a greased baking dish. Let rise again until slightly puffy.
4. **Bake:** Bake in a preheated oven at 375°F (190°C) for 25-30 minutes or until golden brown.
5. **Icing:** made with powdered sweetener, a splash of almond milk, and a touch of rum extract.

Nutritional Values (per roll):

- Calories: 230
- Carbohydrates: 35g
- Protein: 5g
- Fat: 10g
- Sodium: 180mg
- Fiber: 3g

Cooking Tips:

- If using canned pineapple, drain it very well to prevent the rolls from becoming soggy.
- Toast the coconut before adding to the filling for a deeper flavor.

Recipe 66: Chocolate & Cherry Indulgence

Prep Time: 30 mins (+ dough rising time) | **Cook Time:** 25-30 mins

Ingredients:

Sourdough Cinnamon Roll Dough:

- 1 cup sourdough discard (any starter will work)
- 1/2 cup warm water
- 1/4 cup unsweetened almond milk (or other low-carb milk)
- 1 large egg
- 1 tablespoon melted coconut oil or butter.
- 1/4 cup granulated sweetener of choice (monk fruit, stevia, etc.)
- 1/2 teaspoon vanilla extract
- 1 teaspoon baking powder
- 1/2 teaspoon salt
- 2-2 1/2 cups all-purpose flour

Filling:

- 1/2 cup chocolate hazelnut spread (look for sugar-free alternatives)
- 1/4 cup chopped dried cherries.

Alternative Ingredients

- Use other dried fruits instead of cherries, like cranberries or raisins.
- Substitute the chocolate hazelnut spread with other nut butter or a sugar-free chocolate spread.

Step-by-Step Instructions:

1. **Make Sourdough Dough:** Combine sourdough discard, water, almond milk, egg, melted coconut oil, sweetener, vanilla, baking powder, and salt. Gradually add flour until a dough forms. Knead until smooth and elastic. Let rise in a warm place until doubled in size.
2. **Fill & Roll:** Roll out the dough into a rectangle. Spread chocolate hazelnut spread evenly, leaving a small border. Sprinkle with chopped dried cherries. Roll up tightly, seal the edge, and cut into rolls. Place in a greased baking dish. Let rise again until slightly puffy.
3. **Bake:** Bake in a preheated oven at 375°F (190°C) for 25-30 minutes or until golden brown.

Nutritional Values (per roll):

- Calories: 280
- Carbohydrates: 35g
- Protein: 6g
- Fat: 15g
- Sodium: 200mg
- Fiber: 4g

Cooking Tips:

- Warm the chocolate hazelnut spread slightly to make it easier to spread on the dough.
- If you don't have chopped dried cherries, you can roughly chop whole dried cherries.

Chapter 15: Sourdough Biscuits (5 Recipes)

Welcome to "Sourdough Biscuits," a delightful chapter dedicated to exploring the versatility of sourdough through the comforting and familiar form of biscuits. In this chapter, we dive into a variety of biscuit recipes that incorporate sourdough discard, transforming what might otherwise be wasted into warm, fluffy, and flavorful treats. Each recipe is designed to showcase how sourdough can enhance the texture and flavor of biscuits, making them perfect for any time of day, from hearty breakfasts to satisfying snacks.

Sourdough discard adds a depth of flavor and a tender crumb to the traditional biscuit, infusing each bite with the slight tanginess for which sourdough is famed. These recipes also highlight the adaptability of sourdough biscuits, incorporating an array of add-ins from savory to sweet, ensuring there's a biscuit to suit every palate.

Explore the Biscuit Varieties:

- **Recipe 67: Chicken & Herb Biscuits** These savory biscuits blend shredded chicken with fresh rosemary and thyme, creating a perfect match for Dijon mustard. Ideal for brunch or as a side to a hearty soup, these biscuits bring comfort food to new heights.

- **Recipe 68: Ham & Cheddar Drop Biscuits** Packed with chunks of ham and rich cheddar cheese and spiced up with a dash of hot sauce, these biscuits are a delightful savory treat. The addition of amaranth starter adds a subtle complexity that enhances the overall flavor.

- **Recipe 69: Sweet Potato & Pecan Biscuits** Sweet potatoes and pecans make these biscuits sweet and nutty, with maple syrup and cinnamon adding a warm, comforting sweetness. Perfect for a fall breakfast or as a holiday side dish, these biscuits are a sweet twist on the classic.

- **Recipe 70: Spiced Carrot & Raisin Biscuits** With grated carrots, raisins, and a mix of warm spices, these biscuits are reminiscent of carrot cake. The brown rice starter adds a slight nuttiness, making it ideal for a snack or a quick breakfast on the go.

- **Recipe 71: Pumpkin Seed & Cranberry Delight** Celebrate the flavors of fall with pumpkin seeds and dried cranberries mixed into sourdough biscuit dough. Sweetened with a touch of honey, these biscuits are a festive and tasty treat perfect for the holiday season or as a delightful afternoon snack.

Sourdough Discard: A Culinary Asset

In addition to providing mouth-watering recipes, this chapter serves as a guide to using sourdough discard effectively, ensuring that you maximize the potential of every batch of sourdough starter. You'll learn tips for storing and refreshing sourdough discard, along with creative ideas for incorporating it into various types of biscuit dough.

Join us in the pages of "Sourdough Biscuits" to discover new ways to enjoy your sourdough starter and bring a touch of homemade comfort to your table with biscuits that are anything but ordinary. Whether you're a seasoned baker or new to the world of sourdough, these recipes will inspire you to bake, share, and indulge in the rich flavors that only sourdough can provide.

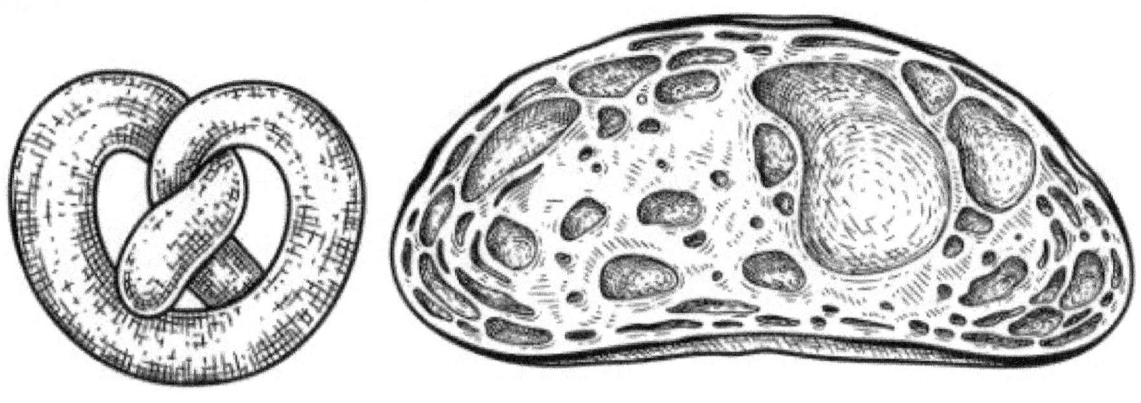

Use a Proofing Basket for Shape and Texture: "Consider using a proofing basket (banneton) to help your sourdough maintain its shape during the final rise and to impart a beautiful pattern on the crust."

Recipe 67: Chicken & Herb Biscuits

Prep Time: 20 mins (+ dough chilling time) | **Cook Time:** 15-20 mins.

Ingredients:

- 2 cups all-purpose flour
- 1 teaspoon baking powder
- 1/2 teaspoon baking soda
- 1/2 teaspoon salt
- 1/4 teaspoon black pepper
- 1 cup cold sourdough discard (any starter will work)
- 1/2 cup cold unsalted butter, cubed.
- 1 cup shredded cooked chicken.
- 2 tablespoons chopped fresh herbs (rosemary, thyme, or a mix)
- 1 tablespoon Dijon mustard
    - 1/4 cup buttermilk or heavy cream

Alternative Ingredients

- Use leftover rotisserie chicken for convenience.
- Substitute herbs with your preferred combination.

Step-by-Step Instructions:

1. **Make Dry Ingredients:** In a bowl, whisk together flour, baking powder, baking soda, salt, and pepper.
2. **Cut in Butter:** Cut the cold butter into the dry ingredients using a pastry cutter or your fingers until the mixture resembles coarse crumbs.
3. **Add Sourdough & Chicken:** Stir in the sourdough discard, shredded chicken, herbs, and mustard until just combined.
4. **Add Buttermilk:** Gradually add buttermilk, mixing until a dough forms. Don't overmix.
5. **Chill:** Refrigerate the dough for at least 30 minutes to make it easier to handle.
6. **Bake:** Preheat oven to 450°F (230°C). Drop a spoonful of dough onto a baking sheet lined with parchment paper. Bake for 15-20 minutes, or until golden brown.

Nutritional Values (per biscuit):

- Calories: 250
- Carbohydrates: 25g
- Protein: 12g
- Fat: 14g
- Sodium: 350mg
- Fiber: 2g

Cooking Tips:

- For extra flakiness, use frozen butter and grate it into the flour mixture.
- Don't overwork the dough – this will lead to tough biscuits.

Recipe 68: Ham & Cheddar Drop Biscuits

Prep Time: 15 mins (+ dough chilling time) | **Cook Time:** 15-20 mins.

Ingredients:

- 2 cups all-purpose flour
- 1 teaspoon baking powder
- 1/2 teaspoon baking soda
- 1/2 teaspoon salt
- 1/4 teaspoon black pepper
- 1 cup cold sourdough discard (amaranth starter preferred)
- 1/2 cup cold unsalted butter, cubed.
- 1 cup diced ham.
- 1 cup shredded cheddar cheese
- 1/4 cup buttermilk or heavy cream
- 1-2 teaspoons hot sauce (optional)

Alternative Ingredients

- Use leftover holiday ham or other types of cooked ham.
- Substitute cheddar cheese with your favorite type of shredded cheese.

Step-by-Step Instructions:

1. **Make Dry Ingredients:** In a bowl, whisk together flour, baking powder, baking soda, salt, and pepper.
2. **Cut in Butter:** Cut the cold butter into the dry ingredients using a pastry cutter or your fingers until the mixture resembles coarse crumbs.
3. **Add Sourdough & Mix-ins:** Stir in the sourdough discard, diced ham, shredded cheese, and hot sauce (if using) until just combined.
4. **Add Buttermilk:** Gradually add buttermilk, mixing until a dough forms. Don't overmix.
5. **Chill:** Refrigerate the dough for at least 30 minutes to make it easier to handle.
6. **Bake:** Preheat oven to 450°F (230°C). Drop a spoonful of dough onto a baking sheet lined with parchment paper. Bake for 15-20 minutes, or until golden brown.

Nutritional Values (per biscuit):

- Calories: 280
- Carbohydrates: 25g
- Protein: 10g
- Fat: 18g
- Sodium: 450mg
- Fiber: 2g

Cooking Tips:

- For extra cheesy flavor, sprinkle some shredded cheese on top of the biscuits before baking.
- If you don't have buttermilk, you can make your own by adding a tablespoon of lemon juice or white vinegar to regular milk and letting it sit for 5 minutes.

Recipe 69: Sweet Potato & Pecan (Gluten-Free)

Prep Time: 30 mins (+ dough chilling time) | **Cook Time:** 15-20 mins.

Ingredients:

- 1 cup gluten-free all-purpose flour blend
- 1 teaspoon baking powder
- 1/2 teaspoon baking soda
- 1/2 teaspoon salt
- 1/2 teaspoon ground cinnamon
- 1/4 teaspoon ground nutmeg
- 1 cup cold sourdough discard (any starter will work)
- 1/4 cup cold unsalted butter, cubed (or vegan butter substitute)
- 1/2 cup mashed sweet potato.
- 1/4 cup chopped pecans.
- 2 tablespoons maple syrup
- 1/4 cup buttermilk or unsweetened almond milk

Alternative Ingredients

- Use walnuts or other nuts in place of pecans.
- Substitute maple syrup with honey or agave nectar.

Step-by-Step Instructions:

1. **Make Dry Ingredients:** In a bowl, whisk together gluten-free flour, baking powder, baking soda, salt, cinnamon, and nutmeg.
2. **Cut in Butter:** Cut the cold butter (or vegan butter) into the dry ingredients using a pastry cutter or your fingers until the mixture resembles coarse crumbs.
3. **Add Sourdough & Mix-ins:** Stir in the sourdough discard, mashed sweet potato, chopped pecans, and maple syrup until just combined.
4. **Add Buttermilk:** Gradually add buttermilk, mixing until a dough forms. Don't overmix.
5. **Chill:** Refrigerate the dough for at least 30 minutes to make it easier to handle.
6. **Bake:** Preheat oven to 425°F (220°C). Drop a spoonful of dough onto a baking sheet lined with parchment paper. Bake for 15-20 minutes, or until golden brown.

Nutritional Values (per biscuit):

- Calories: 200
- Carbohydrates: 30g
- Protein: 4g
- Fat: 10g
- Sodium: 250mg
- Fiber: 3g

Cooking Tips:

- Cook and mash the sweet potato ahead of time to save time.
- Make sure your gluten-free flour blend contains xanthan gum, which helps provide structure to gluten-free baked goods.

Recipe 70: Spiced Carrot & Raisin Biscuits (Gluten-Free)

Prep Time: 20 mins (+ dough chilling time) | **Cook Time:** 15-20 mins.

Ingredients:

- 1 cup gluten-free all-purpose flour blend
- 1 teaspoon baking powder
- 1/2 teaspoon baking soda
- 1/2 teaspoon salt
- 1/2 teaspoon ground cinnamon
- 1/4 teaspoon ground ginger
- 1/4 teaspoon ground nutmeg
- 1 cup cold sourdough discard (brown rice starter preferred)
- 1/4 cup cold unsalted butter, cubed (or vegan butter substitute)
- 1/2 cup grated carrots.
- 1/4 cup raisins
- 2 tablespoons maple syrup
- 1/4 cup buttermilk or unsweetened almond milk

Alternative Ingredients

- Use dried cranberries or other dried fruits in place of raisins.
- Add a pinch of ground cloves for extra warmth.

Step-by-Step Instructions:

1. **Make Dry Ingredients:** In a bowl, whisk together gluten-free flour, baking powder, baking soda, salt, cinnamon, ginger, and nutmeg.
2. **Cut in Butter:** Cut the cold butter (or vegan butter) into the dry ingredients using a pastry cutter or your fingers until the mixture resembles coarse crumbs.
3. **Add Sourdough & Mix-ins:** Stir in the sourdough discard, grated carrots, raisins, and maple syrup until just combined.
4. **Add Buttermilk:** Gradually add buttermilk, mixing until a dough forms. Don't overmix.
5. **Chill:** Refrigerate the dough for at least 30 minutes to make it easier to handle.
6. **Bake:** Preheat oven to 425°F (220°C). Drop a spoonful of dough onto a baking sheet lined with parchment paper. Bake for 15-20 minutes, or until golden brown.

Nutritional Values (per biscuit):

- Calories: 180
- Carbohydrates: 30g
- Protein: 4g
- Fat: 8g
- Sodium: 220mg
- Fiber: 3g

Cooking Tips:

- Grate the carrots finely for even distribution throughout the biscuits.
- If the dough seems too dry, add an extra tablespoon or two of buttermilk.

Recipe 71: Pumpkin Seed & Cranberry Delight (Gluten-Free)

Prep Time: 20 mins (+ dough chilling time) | **Cook Time:** 15-20 mins.

Ingredients:

- 1 cup gluten-free all-purpose flour blend
- 1 teaspoon baking powder
- 1/2 teaspoon baking soda
- 1/2 teaspoon salt
- 1/2 teaspoon ground cinnamon
- 1 cup cold sourdough discard (any starter will work)
- 1/4 cup cold unsalted butter, cubed (or vegan butter substitute)
- 1/4 cup pumpkin seeds
- 1/4 cup dried cranberries
- 2 tablespoons honey
  - 1/4 cup buttermilk or unsweetened almond milk

Alternative Ingredients

- Use sunflower seeds or other nuts in place of pumpkin seeds.
- Substitute dried cranberries with other dried fruits like cherries or blueberries.

Step-by-Step Instructions:

1. **Make Dry Ingredients:** In a bowl, whisk together gluten-free flour, baking powder, baking soda, salt, and cinnamon.
2. **Cut in Butter:** Cut the cold butter (or vegan butter) into the dry ingredients using a pastry cutter or your fingers until the mixture resembles coarse crumbs.
3. **Add Sourdough & Mix-ins:** Stir in the sourdough discard, pumpkin seeds, dried cranberries, and honey until just combined.
4. **Add Buttermilk:** Gradually add buttermilk, mixing until a dough forms. Don't overmix.
5. **Chill:** Refrigerate the dough for at least 30 minutes to make it easier to handle.
6. **Bake:** Preheat oven to 425°F (220°C). Drop a spoonful of dough onto a baking sheet lined with parchment paper. Bake for 15-20 minutes, or until golden brown.

Nutritional Values (per biscuit):

- Calories: 200
- Carbohydrates: 28g
- Protein: 5g
- Fat: 10g
- Sodium: 230mg
- Fiber: 3g

Cooking Tips:

- Toast the pumpkin seeds before adding them to the dough for an extra layer of flavor.
- If you don't have honey, maple syrup can be used as a substitute.

Chapter 16: Creative Leftover Uses (5 Recipes)

Welcome to "Creative Leftover Uses," a chapter dedicated to transforming leftover sourdough bread into delightful culinary creations. This chapter celebrates the versatility and enduring appeal of sourdough by showcasing how to give your day-old bread a delicious second life. Whether you have a few slices or an entire loaf that's past its prime, these recipes provide innovative and tasty solutions to reduce food waste and enjoy sourdough in completely new ways.

Sourdough's unique tang and sturdy texture make it an ideal candidate for repurposing, and each recipe in this chapter is designed to enhance these characteristics, ensuring that nothing goes to waste. From sweet breakfast options to savory dinner dishes, you'll discover how to incorporate leftover sourdough into your meals, turning what might have been discarded into dishes that are both satisfying and environmentally conscious.

Delightful Dishes from Leftover Sourdough:

- **Recipe 72: French Toast Extravaganza** Revive stale sourdough by soaking it in a rich egg custard flavored with flaxseeds, cinnamon, and vanilla. Top the golden-browned slices with fresh berries and a dollop of Greek yogurt for a luxurious breakfast treat.

- **Recipe 73: Gourmet Grilled Cheese** Elevate the classic grilled cheese by using sourdough slices filled with a blend of sharp cheddar and mozzarella, enriched with sautéed mushrooms and caramelized onions for a gourmet touch.

- **Recipe 74: Panzanella Powerhouse** Transform sourdough bread cubes into the star of this robust salad, combining them with grilled chicken, fresh vegetables, feta, and olives, all dressed in a zesty sourdough-infused vinaigrette for a filling and flavorful meal.

- **Recipe 75: Sourdough Bread Pudding** Create a comforting dessert or brunch item by baking chunks of sourdough with nuts, dried fruits, and a cinnamon-spiced custard. This bread pudding is a sweet way to use up larger quantities of leftover bread.

- **Recipe 76: Savory Croutons** Convert sourdough bread into crispy, flavorful croutons by tossing cubes with olive oil, grated Parmesan, Italian herbs, and a touch of sourdough discard. Bake until they are golden and crunchy, perfect for topping salads or soups.

Making the Most of Sourdough

This chapter not only provides you with delicious recipes but also offers tips and tricks for storing and refreshing sourdough to extend its life. You'll learn how the slightly sour and hearty nature of sourdough bread makes it a versatile base for a variety of culinary uses, from enhancing the texture of a dish to adding a layer of flavor complexity.

Join us in embracing sustainability and creativity in the kitchen as we explore the endless possibilities with leftover sourdough. "Creative Leftover Uses" encourages you to look at your breadbox not as a space for forgotten food but as a source of inspiration for your next delicious meal. Whether you're a novice baker or a sourdough enthusiast, this chapter promises to change how you think about and use leftover bread in your culinary adventures.

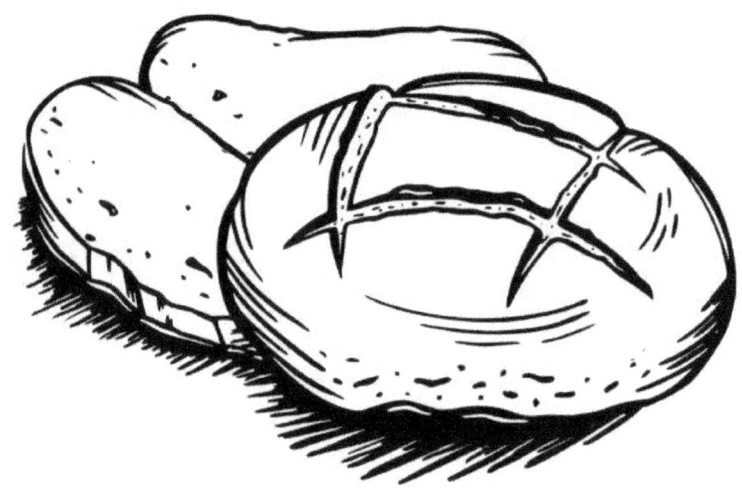

Score Your Dough: "Scoring (cutting) the dough just before baking helps control the direction in which the bread expands and prevents it from bursting at undesirable points. It also enhances the aesthetic of your loaf."

Recipe 72: French Toast Extravaganza

Prep Time: 10 mins | **Cook Time:** 10-15 mins

Ingredients:

Bread: 4-6 thick slices of stale sourdough bread

Egg Custard:

- 2 large eggs
- 1/4 cup milk (or dairy-free alternatives like almond milk, soy milk, etc.)
- 2 tablespoons ground flaxseeds
- 1 teaspoon ground cinnamon
- 1 teaspoon vanilla extract
- 1-2 tablespoons maple syrup (optional, adjust to taste)

For Cooking:

- Butter or cooking oil (coconut oil and avocado oil are good choices)

Toppings:

- Fresh berries (blueberries, raspberries, strawberries, etc.)
- Greek yogurt (or plant-based alternative)
- Maple syrup or honey

Step-by-Step Instructions:

1. **Make the Custard:** In a shallow dish or bowl, whisk together eggs, milk, ground flaxseeds, cinnamon, vanilla extract, and maple syrup (if using). Whisk until well combined.
2. **Soak the Bread:** Dip each slice of sourdough bread into the egg custard, coating both sides evenly. Allow the bread to soak for a few minutes, ensuring it absorbs the flavorful custard. (The longer you soak, the creamier the French toast will be).
3. **Cook the French Toast:** Heat a large skillet or griddle over medium heat. Melt a bit of butter or add a drizzle of cooking oil to the pan. Carefully place the soaked bread slices onto the heated skillet. Cook for 3-5 minutes per side or until golden brown and cooked through. (If the pan gets too hot, reduce the heat slightly).
4. **Serve:** Plate the cooked French toast slices. Top with your favorite toppings – fresh berries, a dollop of Greek yogurt, a drizzle of maple syrup, or honey.
5. Enjoy immediately!

Nutritional Values (per 2 slices):

- Calories: 300-400 (depending on toppings and amount of butter/oil used)
- Carbohydrates: 35-45g
- Protein: 15-20g
- Fat: 15-20g
- Sodium: 200-300mg
- Fiber: 4-6g

Cooking Tips:

- Staler bread soaks up more custard, resulting in creamier French toast, but fresh bread works too!
- Add a pinch of nutmeg or cardamom to the custard mixture for extra warmth and spice.

Recipe 73: Gourmet Grilled Cheese

Prep Time: 10 mins | **Cook Time:** 10-15 mins

Ingredients:

Bread:

- 4 slices of sourdough bread

Cheese:

- 1/2 cup shredded sharp cheddar cheese.
- 1/4 cup shredded mozzarella cheese

Fillings:

- 1-2 tablespoons sauteed mushrooms (sliced white or cremini mushrooms work well)
- 1-2 tablespoons caramelized onions

For Cooking:

- Butter (or vegan butter substitute)

Step-by-Step Instructions:

Prepare Fillings (if needed):

1. **Sautéed Mushrooms:** If not already prepared, heat a bit of olive oil in a pan over medium heat. Add sliced mushrooms and cook until softened and slightly browned. Season with salt and pepper.
2. **Caramelized Onions:** If not already prepared, thinly slice an onion and cook it slowly in a bit of olive oil over low heat until soft and deeply golden brown (this can take 20-30 minutes).

Assemble the Sandwiches:

3. Lightly butter one side of each slice of sourdough bread.
4. Place two slices of bread, buttered side down, on a cutting board, skillet, or griddle.
5. Top each slice with a layer of shredded cheddar cheese, followed by a layer of mozzarella cheese.
6. Distribute the sautéed mushrooms and caramelized onions evenly over the cheese.
7. Place the remaining two slices of bread, buttered side up, on top of the sandwiches.

Grill:

8. Heat a skillet or griddle over medium heat.
9. Carefully transfer the assembled sandwiches to the heated surface.
10. Cook for 3-5 minutes per side, or until the bread is golden brown crispy, and the cheese is melted and gooey. (You may need to gently press down on the sandwiches with a spatula to help them cook evenly).
11. Serve:
12. Remove the grilled cheese sandwiches from the heat and let them rest for a minute before cutting them in half.
13. Enjoy immediately while the cheese is still warm and melty!

Nutritional Values (per sandwich):

- ❖ Calories: 450-550 (depending on the amount of butter and cheese used)
- ❖ Carbohydrates: 40-50g
- ❖ Protein: 25-35g
- ❖ Fat: 25-35g
- ❖ Sodium: 600-800mg
- ❖ Fiber: 3-5g

Cooking Tips:

- ✓ Use a mix of cheeses for the best flavor and melt.
- ✓ For extra caramelization, add a pinch of sugar to the onions while they cook.

Recipe 74: Panzanella Powerhouse

Prep Time: 20 mins | **Cook Time:** 10 mins (for grilling chicken)

Ingredients:

Bread:

- 3-4 cups cubed sourdough bread (about 1-inch cubes), slightly stale, is best.

Grilled Chicken:

- 1-2 boneless, skinless chicken breasts

Vegetables:

- 1 large tomato, chopped.
- 1 cucumber, sliced.
- 1/2 cup crumbled feta cheese
- 1/4 cup kalamata olives, pitted and halved.

Vinaigrette:

- 1/4 cup olive oil
- 2 tablespoons sourdough discard
- 2 tablespoons red wine vinegar (or lemon juice)
- 1 teaspoon dried oregano
- 1/2 teaspoon Dijon mustard
- Salt and pepper to taste

Optional Additions:

- Other vegetables like bell peppers, red onion, or artichoke hearts.
- Fresh herbs like basil or parsley.

Step-by-Step Instructions:

1. Grill the Chicken:
2. Season chicken breasts with salt, pepper, and any desired spices (garlic powder, paprika, etc.).
3. Grill or pan-sear the chicken over medium-high heat until cooked through (internal temperature reaches 165°F). Let cool, and then slice or shred the chicken.
4. Toast the Bread (optional):
5. If desired, toast the cubed sourdough bread in a skillet with a bit of olive oil until lightly golden and crisp.
6. Make the Vinaigrette:
7. In a small jar or bowl, whisk together olive oil, sourdough discard, red wine vinegar, dried oregano, Dijon mustard, salt, and pepper.
8. Assemble the Salad:
9. In a large bowl, combine sourdough bread, grilled chicken, tomato, cucumber, feta cheese, and kalamata olives.
10. Drizzle vinaigrette over the salad and toss to coat.
11. Let the salad sit for a few minutes to allow the bread to soak up the dressing.

Nutritional Values (per serving):

- Calories: 400-500 (depending on the amount of chicken and dressing used)
- Carbohydrates: 30-40g
- Protein: 30-40g
- Fat: 20-30g
- Sodium: 500-700mg
- Fiber: 5-8g

Cooking Tips:

- ✓ Don't overdress the salad initially. You can always add more vinaigrette before serving.
- ✓ If you don't have grilled chicken, use rotisserie chicken or leftover cooked chicken.

Recipe 75: Sourdough Bread Pudding

Prep Time: 15 mins | **Cook Time:** 35-45 mins

Ingredients:

Bread:

- 3-4 cups cubed sourdough bread (about 1-inch cubes), slightly stale

Custard:

- 2 large eggs
- 1 cup unsweetened almond milk (or other low-calorie milk)
- 1/4 cup granulated sweetener of choice (monk fruit, stevia, or sugar)
- 1 teaspoon ground cinnamon
- 1/2 teaspoon vanilla extract
- 1/4 teaspoon nutmeg

Additions:

- 1/2 cup chopped walnuts or pecans.
- 1/2 cup raisins or other dried fruit (cranberries, chopped dates)

Optional Toppings:

- Light whipped cream or yogurt
- A sprinkle of cinnamon

Alternative Ingredients:

- For a richer custard, you can use whole milk or a mix of milk and cream.
- Substitute or mix in a variety of nuts and dried fruits to your liking.

Step-by-Step Instructions:

1. Preheat Oven & Prep Bread:
2. Preheat oven to 350°F (175°C).
3. Grease a 9x13-inch baking dish.
4. Arrange the cubed sourdough bread in the prepared baking dish.
5. Make the Custard:
6. In a bowl, whisk together eggs, almond milk, sweetener, cinnamon, vanilla extract, and nutmeg.
7. Combine & Bake:
8. Add chopped nuts and dried fruit (if using) to the bread in the baking dish.
9. Pour the custard mixture over the bread, ensuring it's evenly coated.
10. Bake for 35-45 minutes or until the pudding is set and golden brown. (A knife inserted in the center should come out clean).
11. Serve:
12. Let the bread pudding cool slightly before serving.
13. Top with a dollop of light whipped cream or yogurt and a sprinkle of cinnamon, if desired.

Nutritional Values (per serving):

- Calories: 250-300 (depending on toppings)
- Carbohydrates: 35-45g
- Protein: 10-12g
- Fat: 12-15g
- Sodium: 150-200mg
- Fiber: 4-6g

Cooking Tips:

- Ensure the bread cubes are stale or lightly toasted to help absorb the custard without becoming soggy.
- Let the bread pudding soak in the custard mixture for at least 10-15 minutes before baking for optimal flavor and texture.

Recipe 76: Savory Croutons

Prep Time: 10 mins | **Cook Time:** 15-20 mins.

Ingredients:

Bread:

- 3-4 cups cubed sourdough bread (about 1-inch cubes), slightly stale.

Flavorings:

- 1/4 cup olive oil
- 1/4 cup grated parmesan cheese.
- 1 tablespoon dried Italian herbs (or herb blend of your choice)
- 1 teaspoon garlic powder
- 1/4 teaspoon sourdough discard (optional, adds a subtle tang)
- Salt and pepper to taste

Alternative Ingredients:

- Substitute Parmesan cheese with other grated hard cheeses like Asiago or Romano.
- Play around with different spices – try adding smoked paprika, a pinch of red pepper flakes, or some Cajun seasoning.

Step-by-Step Instructions:

1. **Preheat oven:** Preheat oven to 375°F (190°C). Line a baking sheet with parchment paper.
2. **Toss with Flavorings:** In a large bowl, combine the cubed sourdough bread with olive oil, parmesan cheese, dried herbs, garlic powder, sourdough discard (if using), salt, and pepper. Toss until the bread cubes are evenly coated.
3. **Bake:** Spread the seasoned bread cubes in a single layer on the prepared baking sheet. Bake for 15-20 minutes or until golden brown and crispy, stirring occasionally to even browning.
4. **Cool & Store:** Let the croutons cool completely on the baking sheet. Store in an airtight container at room temperature for up to a week.

Nutritional Values (per 1/4 cup serving):

- ❖ Calories: 120-150
- ❖ Carbohydrates: 10-12g
- ❖ Protein: 4-5g
- ❖ Fat: 8-10g
- ❖ Sodium: 200-250mg
- ❖ Fiber: 1-2g

Cooking Tips:

- ✓ The size of your bread cubes will affect the baking time, so adjust accordingly if you cut them smaller or larger.
- ✓ For extra crispness, turn off the oven after cooking time and let the croutons cool inside the oven.

Chapter 17: Advanced Techniques & Flavor Exploration

Look, a rustic, cracked loaf is gorgeous in its own way. But sometimes, you wanna step it up, right? We're talking about tight boules, perfectly scored batards, and those braided beauties that make people ask where the heck you bought your bread.

Shaping Beautiful Loaves: Step Up Your Bread Game

Forget those unintentionally lopsided loaves – we're going pro! Shaping sourdough is about more than aesthetics; it builds a structure for the perfect crumb, that airy, holey goodness with a satisfying chew.

Here's what you'll master:

- **Stretch & Fold:** This isn't aggressive kneading. It's a gentle technique where you repeatedly stretch and fold the dough, building gluten strength. Strong gluten means your dough will hold its shape and rise beautifully.
- **Wet Your Hands:** Slightly damp hands help prevent the dough from sticking.
- **Grab & Stretch:** Reach under one side of your dough and gently lift a large section. Stretch it upwards as much as possible without tearing.
- **Fold It Over:** Fold the stretched section of dough over the center of your loaf.
- **Rotate & Repeat:** Turn your bowl or container 90 degrees and repeat the stretch and fold process from this new side.
- **Keep On Folding:** Continue rotating and repeating the stretches and folds around the dough about 4-6 times total.

Why Does it Work?

- **Gluten Development:** Each stretch strengthens those gluten strands, making your dough more elastic and giving it the ability to hold its shape.
- **Structure:** The folding action helps distribute gas bubbles from the yeast throughout the dough, leading to an even rise.

- **Shaping Control:** A strong, well-developed dough is easier to handle and shape without deflating.

Tips:

- **Rest Periods:** Allow the dough to rest for 20-30 minutes between sets of stretch and folds. This gives the gluten-free time to relax, making the stretching easier.
- **Be Gentle:** Avoid overworking the dough. Handle it gently to prevent tearing.
- **Watch & Learn:** There are tons of great videos online demonstrating the stretch and fold technique. Seeing it in action can be very helpful!
- **Building Tension:** Imagine a taught drumhead. That's the kind of surface we want on our dough. By gently pulling and folding the dough during shaping, we create a tight surface that allows for a spectacular rise in the oven and helps those decorative scores (cuts) open cleanly.

Building Tension in Sourdough Shaping: A Step-by-Step Guide

1. Shaping Techniques:

- **Stretch and Fold:** During this technique, you gently stretch the dough upwards and fold it over itself. This creates layers and aligns the gluten strands, which are responsible for the structure.
- **Rounding:** After several stretches and folds, you'll gently shape the dough into a ball. Imagine cupping your hands around the dough and moving them in a circular motion, coaxing the dough into a smooth, round shape. Use a light touch and avoid overworking the dough.
- **Surface Tension:** As you round the dough, focus on creating a smooth, taught surface. Imagine gently pulling the dough upwards and inwards with your fingertips, almost like tightening a drawstring on a bag.

2. Visual and Tactile Cues:

- **Look:** After rounding, the dough surface should appear smooth and slightly taut. It shouldn't be loose or floppy, but it shouldn't be rock-hard, either.
- **Touch:** Gently press your fingertip on the surface. It should feel slightly firm and spring back a little when you release it. This "bounce" indicates good tension.

3. Benefits of Tension:

- **Oven Spring:** The tight surface holds in the gas produced by the yeast during baking. This allows for a dramatic rise, creating a beautiful oven spring.

- **Cleaner Scores:** When you score the top of your dough before baking, a tight surface allows the cuts to open cleanly. This controlled release of steam contributes to a good rise.
- **Improved Crumb:** Tension helps distribute the gas bubbles evenly throughout the dough. This results in a more uniform crumb with desirable air pockets and a satisfying chew.

4. **Tips:**

- **Practice Makes Perfect:** Building tension takes practice. As you get comfortable with shaping techniques, you'll develop a feel for the right amount of tension.
- **Be Gentle:** Remember, we're aiming for taut, not tight. Overworking the dough can damage the gluten strands and hinder the rise.
- **Visual and Tactile Cues:** Rely on both your eyes and fingertips to assess the tension. A smooth, slightly firm surface with a little "bounce" is what you're aiming for.

With experience, you might even hear a slight popping sound when gently pressing dough with good tension. This sound indicates the gluten strands stretching and aligning.

- **Braiding & Beyond:** Now it is fun! We'll move past basic rounds and explore shaping techniques for stunning loaves. Think classic batards (oblong loaves), beautiful boules (round loaves), and even impressive braids that will have everyone asking where you bought your bread (it'll be your secret!).

STEP-BY-STEP GUIDE

1. Batards: The Sleek Classic

- What it is: An oblong-shaped loaf with gently tapered ends.
- How to: After initial shaping (stretch and fold, rounding), gently roll the dough out into a rectangle. Fold one-third of the dough towards the center, then fold the other third over it like a letter. Finally, seal the seam by gently rolling the dough over.

2. Boules: Rustic Elegance

- What it is: A perfectly round loaf, the ultimate test of shaping skill.
- How to: After shaping into a ball, use your cupped hands to create even tension on the surface. Move your hands gently around the dough ball, pulling the surface slightly inwards. Continue rotating until the dough feels smooth and taut.

3. Braids: The Showstopper

- What it is: Interwoven strands of dough, perfect for showcasing variations with seeds, spices, or even colorful fillings.
- How to: Divide your dough into 3-6 strands (depending on the braid complexity you want). Roll each strand into a long rope. Braid the strands, tucking the ends neatly underneath.

Important Notes:

- YouTube to the Rescue: Search for "(shaping technique name) sourdough" on YouTube for visual demonstrations. Seeing it in action is incredibly helpful!
- It's a Learning Curve: Don't worry if your first attempts aren't perfect. Each loaf teaches you something about the dough and your technique.
- Get Creative: Braids can be done with sweet doughs, filled with chocolate or marzipan, savory with pesto and cheese...let your imagination run wild!

The sky's the limit! Explore intricate scoring patterns, swirls of different colors and flavors in your dough, and knotted bread...your sourdough journey is only getting more exciting!

Beyond These Basics:

Whole Grains & Seeds: Flavor & Nutrition Powerhouses

Listen, refined white flour is all fine and predictable, but it's a nutritional snooze-fest. Think of whole grains and seeds like the rock stars of baking – they're bold, packed with flavor, and surprisingly good for you. Spelt, with its nutty sweetness, the earthy depth of rye, the satisfying chew of oats... these guys bring the party! Plus, those little bursts of poppy seeds and pumpkin seeds are like adding edible confetti.

The Catch: Think Different.

Whole grains and seeds aren't like your basic white flour. They're different beasts, and we need to shift our approach. Here's what you need to know:

- **Hydration is Key:** Whole grains are THIRSTY. They soak up more water than refined flour. We'll master adjusting our dough hydration to get the perfect texture without turning your loaf into a brick.

- **Soakers & Sprouters:** This is next-level stuff. By soaking or sprouting our grains and seeds, we unlock hidden nutrients, improve digestibility, and coax out even more intense flavor. It's a little extra effort, but trust me, it's worth it.

- **Mix & Match Magic:** We're not just substituting whole grains one-for-one. I'll teach you about perfect pairings for flavor and texture. A touch of spelt for sweetness. Rye for a complex depth? Rolled oats for chew? We'll find your favorite combos, and a hint of honey or maple syrup can bring it all together.

Get Ready: Your sourdough is about to get a whole lot more flavorful, nutritious, and interesting. Ditch the boring, and let's go on a whole-grain adventure!

Naturally Sweetened Sourdough

Bakers, let's talk about adding a subtle touch of sweetness to your sourdough game. Think of it as the elegant cousin, not the sugar-bomb nephew, of your classic tangy loaves. This isn't about making dessert bread; it's about unlocking those delicate sweet notes and creating something truly special.

Here's how we'll play with natural sweetness:

- Fruity Ferments: Forget plain old water and flour! We're going to feed our starters dried fruits, mashed ripe bananas, and even fruit juices. This infuses the starter itself with a gentle sweetness and complex flavor.
- Spice is Nice: Forget cinnamon swirls! We're using spices strategically, highlighting their warm, sweet qualities without being overwhelming. Think ginger for a little bit, cardamom for a floral touch, or a combination that's uniquely yours.
- The Power of Malt: This ingredient might be new to you, but trust me – it's our secret weapon! Malt adds a subtle sweetness, a touch of that toasty caramel flavor, and helps with a beautiful crust.

Here's Why This Matters:

- Balance: A hint of sweetness beautifully offsets the sourdough tang, creating a layered flavor experience.
- Versatility: These breads aren't just for dessert! They're amazing for special breakfast spreads, paired with cheeses, or as the base for savory toasts.
- Subtly Unique: This isn't about replicating store-bought cinnamon bread. You're going to create a nuanced, sophisticated sweetness that has your own signature.
- Seasonal Flavor Inspiration

Lastly, let's ditch the predictable flavors and embrace the wild, seasonal side of sourdough! It's about using nature as your inspiration, your grocery list, and baking masterpieces that change as the world around you blooms, ripens, and grows.

Here's the chef's take on seasonal baking:

- Freshness is Key: Don't settle for out-of-season, flavorless imports. We're baking with the freshest produce at its peak flavor. Think delicate spring herbs that sing in a loaf, juicy summer berries bursting through your crumb, or roasted autumn vegetables bringing warmth to your table.

- Celebrate the Seasons: Baking shouldn't feel static. Imagine the thrill of those first spring loaves with hints of chives or that rhubarb swirl. Picture sourdough pizzas on the patio adorned with summer's bounty. Then, the comforting warmth of pumpkin spice (yes, when it's used right!), followed by festive winter bread with cranberries and citrus.

- It's About More Than Recipes: Seasonal sourdough baking is about creativity, resourcefulness, and a connection to the changing year. You're tapping into nature's rhythms, showcasing the local, the delicious, and making sourdough a living, breathing art.

Let's break it down:

- Spring: Think fresh, vibrant flavors – herbal loaves, lemony starters, maybe a wild ramp twist if you're lucky.

- Summer: Explosion of color and flavor – sourdough pizzas piled high, bright berry swirls, maybe even a grilled peach and goat cheese focaccia.

- Autumn: Warmth and richness take center stage – apples, nuts, earthy spices, and yes, pumpkin done with a sophisticated hand.

- Winter: Cozy and festive – citrus for brightness, cranberries for tartness, spiced bread pudding, turning your stale sourdough into a comforting treat.

Chapter 18: Accompaniments for Your Sourdough

Welcome to "Accompaniments for Your Sourdough," where we explore a delightful array of dishes specifically designed to complement the robust flavors and textures of sourdough bread. This chapter is a treasure trove for those who cherish their sourdough and seek to enhance their experience with perfectly paired side dishes and accompaniments. Whether you're a sourdough enthusiast or just starting to explore the versatility of this artisan bread, these recipes will inspire you to create harmonious pairings that elevate your meals.

Sourdough bread, with its distinctively tangy flavor and chewy texture, serves as more than just a side—it's a foundational element that can transform a simple meal into an extraordinary culinary event. The recipes in this chapter are crafted to match the character of sourdough, from the simplest spreads to more elaborate side dishes, ensuring that every bite is as satisfying as it is delicious.

Crafting the Perfect Pairings

Each recipe in this chapter not only complements sourdough but also enhances it, allowing the unique flavors of the bread to shine through while providing a balanced and enriching culinary experience. Here's a preview of what to expect:

- Savory Spreads: Discover a variety of spreads from rich and creamy to bright and tangy, each designed to spread beautifully on a slice of toasted sourdough.

- Elegant Olives and Tapenades: Dive into the world of marinated olives and rustic tapenades that bring a Mediterranean flair to your sourdough, perfect for an elevated snack or a sophisticated appetizer.

- Cheese Pairings: Learn how to pair different types of cheese with sourdough, from soft and creamy to hard and mature, creating combinations that please the palate.

- Homemade Jams and Jellies: Explore sweet accompaniments like fig jam or blackberry jelly that contrast wonderfully with the sour notes of sourdough, ideal for breakfast or a decadent snack.

- Vegetable Sides: Enjoy recipes for roasted, sautéed, or raw vegetables that complement the hearty attributes of sourdough, making for a balanced meal or a wholesome brunch.

The Joy of Sourdough

As you delve into the recipes of "Accompaniments for Your Sourdough," you'll gain a deeper appreciation for the versatility of sourdough bread. This chapter encourages culinary creativity and invites you to experiment with flavors and textures that make each meal with sourdough an exciting adventure.

Prepare to be inspired by the array of possibilities that await in this chapter, as each recipe promises to enhance your dining experience, turning simple sourdough bread into a canvas for culinary artistry. Whether you're hosting a dinner party, enjoying a family meal, or simply indulging in a personal treat, these accompaniments will make your sourdough sing with flavor.

Simple Spreads & Dips (6 Recipes)

Recipe 77: Quinoa & Avocado Hummus: Combine cooked quinoa, avocado, chickpeas, tahini, lemon juice, garlic, a touch of olive oil, and a sprinkle of sourdough discard for a bright and tangy twist.

Recipe 78: Roasted Red Pepper & Feta Dip: Blend roasted red peppers, feta cheese, walnuts, garlic, herbs, a drizzle of olive oil, and a spoonful of sourdough discard for a tangy, Mediterranean-inspired dip.

Recipe 79: White Bean & Spinach Spread: Sautéed spinach, white beans, garlic, lemon zest, a hint of nutritional yeast, and sourdough discard create a creamy and vibrant spread.

Recipe 80: Sundried Tomato & Basil Pesto: Blend sundried tomatoes, fresh basil, pine nuts, garlic, olive oil, and a dollop of sourdough discard. It is delicious on sandwiches or crackers.

Recipe 81: Lentil & Carrot Dip: Cooked lentils, grated carrots, spices (cumin, coriander), tahini, lemon juice, a hint of harissa paste, and sourdough discard form a flavorful and satisfying dip.

Recipe 82: Smoked Paprika & Cashew Cheese: Blend-soaked cashews, nutritional yeast, smoked paprika, garlic, lemon juice, and sourdough discard for a creamy and smoky plant-based "cheese" spread.

Recipe 77: Quinoa & Avocado Hummus

Prep Time: 10 mins (+ quinoa cooking time) | **Servings:** 4-6

Ingredients:

- 1/2 cup cooked quinoa
- 1 ripe avocado
- 1 can (15 oz) chickpeas, drained and rinsed.
- 2 tablespoons tahini
- 2 tablespoons lemon juice
- 1-2 cloves garlic, minced.
- 1/4 cup olive oil
- 1/4 cup sourdough discard (brown rice or sorghum starter is preferable)
- Salt and pepper to taste
- Pinch of cumin (optional)

Best Sourdough Starter: A neutral-flavored starter like brown rice or sorghum works best to blend seamlessly with the other flavors.

Step-by-Step Instructions:

1. **Blend:** Combine all ingredients in a food processor and blend until smooth and creamy. Add a little water if needed to achieve desired consistency.
2. **Adjust Seasoning:** Taste and adjust salt, pepper, and spices as needed.
3. **Serve:** Serve with pita bread, vegetables, or crackers. Garnish with a drizzle of olive oil and a sprinkle of paprika or sumac for an extra touch.

Nutritional Values (per 1/4 cup serving):

- Calories: 180
- Carbohydrates: 20g
- Protein: 8g
- Fat: 10g
- Sodium: 150mg
- Fiber: 6g

Cooking Tips:

- Use pre-cooked or leftover quinoa for convenience.
- If you don't have tahini, substitute with an equal amount of cashew butter or sunflower seed butter.

Special Diets:

- **Vegan**: This recipe is already vegan-friendly!
- **Gluten-free:** Ensure you serve with gluten-free pita bread or crackers.

Recipe 78: Roasted Red Pepper & Feta Dip

Prep Time: 15 mins (+ red pepper roasting time) | **Servings:** 4-6

Ingredients:

- 2 large red bell peppers, roasted, peeled, and seeded.
- 1/2 cup crumbled feta cheese
- 1/4 cup walnuts
- 1-2 cloves garlic, minced.
- 1 tablespoon olive oil
- 2 tablespoons lemon juice
- 1 tablespoon sourdough discard (any variety)
- 1/2 teaspoon dried oregano
- Salt and pepper to taste

Best Sourdough Starter: Any starter will work well here, as the flavors of the roasted peppers and feta will be dominant.

Step-by-Step Instructions:

1. **Roast Peppers:** Roast red bell peppers under a broiler or on a grill until charred and blistered. Let it cool slightly, then peel, seed, and roughly chop.
2. **Blend:** Combine roasted peppers, feta cheese, walnuts, garlic, olive oil, lemon juice, sourdough discard, oregano, salt, and pepper in a food processor. Blend until mostly smooth but slightly chunky.
3. **Adjust Seasoning:** Taste and adjust salt, pepper, and lemon juice as needed.
4. **Serve:** Serve with pita chips, crackers, or fresh vegetables.

Nutritional Values (per 1/4 cup serving):

- Calories: 150
- Carbohydrates: 8g
- Protein: 6g
- Fat: 12g
- Sodium: 300mg
- Fiber: 2g

Cooking Tips:

- Use jarred roasted red peppers for a time-saving shortcut.
- Toast the walnuts before adding them to the food processor for enhanced flavor.
- Garnish with fresh herbs like parsley or basil for a pop of color.

Special Diets:

- **Vegetarian:** This recipe is already vegetarian-friendly!
- **Vegan:** For a vegan version, substitute feta cheese with a vegan alternative or omit.

Recipe 79: White Bean & Spinach Spread

Prep Time: 10 mins | **Servings:** 4-6

Ingredients:

- 1 can (15 oz) white beans (cannellini beans), drained and rinsed.
- 5 ounces baby spinach, sautéed.
- 1-2 cloves garlic, minced.
- 1 tablespoon lemon juice
- 2 tablespoons olive oil
- 1/4 cup sourdough discard (any variety)
- 1/4 cup nutritional yeast (for cheesy flavor)
- Salt and pepper to taste

Best Sourdough Starter: Any starter will work well. The main flavor contributions come from the spinach, lemon, and nutritional yeast.

Alternative Ingredients:

- Substitute white beans with other cooked beans like chickpeas or kidney beans.
- If baby spinach is unavailable, use frozen spinach (thawed and squeezed dry) or other leafy greens like kale or Swiss chard.

Step-by-Step Instructions:

1. **Sauté:** Sauté garlic in a bit of olive oil until fragrant. Add spinach and cook until wilted. Season with a pinch of salt and pepper.
2. **Blend:** Combine white beans, sautéed spinach, lemon juice, olive oil, sourdough discard, nutritional yeast, salt, and pepper in a food processor. Blend until smooth and creamy.
3. **Adjust Seasoning:** Taste and adjust salt, pepper, and lemon juice as needed.
4. **Serve:** Serve with crackers, toasted bread, or as a sandwich spread.

Nutritional Values (per 1/4 cup serving):

- Calories: 160
- Carbohydrates: 20g
- Protein: 8g
- Fat: 7g
- Sodium: 200mg
- Fiber: 6g

Cooking Tips:

- ✓ Squeeze out excess liquid from the spinach after it's cooked to prevent a watery spread.
- ✓ Add a pinch of red pepper flakes for a touch of spice.

Special Diets:

- **Vegan**: This recipe is already vegan-friendly!
- **Gluten-free**: Ensure you serve with gluten-free bread or crackers.

Recipe 80: Sundried Tomato & Basil Pesto

Prep Time: 10 mins | **Cook Time:** None | **Servings:** Makes about 1 cup!

Ingredients:

- 1/2 cup packed sundried tomatoes (not oil-packed)
- 1/2 cup packed fresh basil leaves.
- 1/4 cup pine nuts (or walnuts)
- 2 cloves garlic, minced.
- 1/4 cup olive oil
- 2 tablespoons grated parmesan cheese.
- 2 tablespoons sourdough discard (any variety)
- Salt and pepper to taste

Best Sourdough Starter: Any starter will work – the robust sundried tomato and basil will be the dominant flavors.

Alternative Ingredients:

- To rehydrate sundried tomatoes, soak them in hot water for about 15 minutes.
- Substitute pine nuts with other nuts like almonds or cashews.

Step-by-Step Instructions:

1. **Blend:** Combine sundried tomatoes, basil, nuts, garlic, olive oil, parmesan cheese, and sourdough, and discard them in a food processor. Pulse until a coarse paste forms.
2. **Adjust Seasoning:** Taste and season with salt and pepper as needed.
3. **Serve:** Toss with pasta, spread on sandwiches or pizzas, or use as a dip for vegetables.

Nutritional Values (per 2 tablespoons):

- Calories: 120
- Carbohydrates: 5g
- Protein: 3g
- Fat: 11g
- Sodium: 120mg
- Fiber: 1g

Cooking Tips:

- Toast the pine nuts (or substitute nuts) for a deeper flavor.
- If the pesto is too thick, add a little more olive oil to achieve the desired consistency.
- Store leftover pesto in the refrigerator for up to a week.

Special Diets:

- **Vegetarian**: This recipe is already vegetarian-friendly!
- **Vegan:** For a vegan version, omit the parmesan cheese or substitute it with nutritional yeast.

Recipe 81: Lentil & Carrot Dip

Prep Time: 15 mins (+ lentil cooking time) | **Cook Time:** 20-25 mins (lentils) | **Servings:** 4-6

Ingredients:

- 1/2 cup green or brown lentils
- 1 medium carrot, grated.
- 1/4 cup tahini
- 2 tablespoons lemon juice
- 1 tablespoon olive oil
- 1 clove garlic, minced.
- 1/2 teaspoon cumin
- 1/4 teaspoon coriander
- Pinch of harissa paste (optional for heat)
- 1/4 cup sourdough discard (any variety)
- Salt and pepper to taste

Best Sourdough Starter: Any starter works well here; the spices and other flavors are the stars.

Alternative Ingredients:

- Use other types of cooked lentils, like red lentils (they cook faster).
- Substitute harissa paste with a pinch of cayenne pepper or red pepper flakes.

Step-by-Step Instructions:

1. **Cook Lentils:** Cook lentils according to package directions until tender but not mushy. Drain and set aside.
2. **Blend:** Combine cooked lentils, grated carrot, tahini, lemon juice, olive oil, garlic, cumin, coriander, harissa paste (if using), sourdough discard, salt, and pepper in a food processor. Blend until mostly smooth with a slightly coarse texture.
3. **Adjust Seasoning:** Taste and adjust salt, pepper, lemon juice, and spices as needed.
4. **Serve:** Serve with pita bread, crackers, or fresh vegetables.

Nutritional Values (per 1/4 cup serving):

- Calories: 140
- Carbohydrates: 15g
- Protein: 7g
- Fat: 7g
- Sodium: 120mg
- Fiber: 5g

Cooking Tips:

- ✓ Add chopped fresh herbs like parsley or cilantro for a bright flavor.
- ✓ Garnish with a sprinkle of toasted sesame seeds for a nutty touch.

Special Diets:

- **Vegan:** This recipe is already vegan-friendly!
- **Gluten-free:** Ensure you serve with gluten-free pita bread or crackers.

Recipe 82: Smoked Paprika & Cashew Cheese

Prep Time: 10 mins (+ cashew soaking time) | **Cook Time:** None | **Servings:** Makes about 1 cup

Ingredients:

- 1 cup raw cashews, soaked in water for at least 4 hours or overnight.
- 1/4 cup nutritional yeast
- 1 tablespoon smoked paprika.
- 1 tablespoon lemon juice
- 1 clove garlic, minced.
- 1/4 cup sourdough discard (any variety)
- 1/4 cup water (more or less as needed)
- Salt and pepper to taste

Best Sourdough Starter: A neutral starter like brown rice or sorghum works best to complement the other seasonings.

Alternative Ingredients:

- Substitute smoked paprika with regular paprika or a combination of paprika and a pinch of chipotle powder.

Step-by-Step Instructions:

1. **Soak Cashews:** Soak cashews in water for at least 4 hours or overnight to soften them. Drain and rinse well.
2. **Blend:** Combine soaked cashews, nutritional yeast, smoked paprika, lemon juice, garlic, sourdough discard, water, salt, and pepper in a high-powered blender or food processor. Blend until very smooth and creamy, adding more water if needed for consistency.
3. **Adjust Seasoning:** Taste and adjust salt, pepper, lemon juice, and smoked paprika as needed.
4. **Serve:** Serve with crackers, vegetables, or as a spread on sandwiches.

Nutritional Values (per 2 tablespoons):

- Calories: 100
- Carbohydrates: 6g
- Protein: 5g
- Fat: 7g
- Sodium: 100mg
- Fiber: 1g

Cooking Tips:

- For an extra creamy consistency, add a tablespoon of olive oil.
- Store leftover cashew cheese spread in an airtight container in the refrigerator for up to 5 days.

Special Diets:

- **Vegan:** This recipe is already vegan-friendly!
- **Gluten-free:** Ensure you serve with gluten-free crackers.

Chapter 19: Soups & Stews to Pair with Sourdough (6 Recipes)

Welcome to "Soups & Stews to Pair with Sourdough," a warming chapter of our cookbook that brings together the rustic charm of sourdough bread with the comforting embrace of soups and stews. This chapter is designed to explore the harmonious relationship between freshly baked sourdough and a variety of rich, nourishing soups and stews, each recipe carefully crafted to enhance this classic pairing.

Sourdough bread, known for its tangy flavor and chewy texture, is the perfect complement to the complex flavors of soups and stews. Its sturdy crust and tender crumb make it ideal for dipping and sopping up rich broths, adding a satisfying texture and flavor depth to each spoonful. In this chapter, we delve into recipes that not only warm the soul but also celebrate the versatility of sourdough as more than just a side dish—it's an integral part of the meal, enhancing and absorbing the delicious flavors of the soups and stews.

Explore the Culinary Pairings

Each recipe in this chapter incorporates sourdough in unique ways, from a swirl of sourdough discard that adds body and flavor to creamy soups to chunks of crusty bread that bring texture and heartiness to robust stews. Here's what you can expect:

- **Recipe 83: Creamy Carrot & Quinoa Soup** A silky blend of sautéed carrots and cooked quinoa thickened with sourdough discard for an extra creamy texture, making every bite a delightful experience.

- **Recipe 84: Hearty Lentil & Kale Stew** Dive into the rustic flavors of lentils and kale stewed with tomatoes and a base enriched with sourdough discard, offering a hearty and fulfilling dish perfect for chilly evenings.

- **Recipe 85: Tomato & White Bean Bisque** A smooth and creamy bisque where the mild flavors of white beans and roasted tomatoes are enhanced by the unique addition of sourdough discard, providing a subtle tang and richness.

- **Recipe 86: Spiced Butternut Squash & Chickpea Soup** Enjoy the sweet and spicy blend of roasted butternut squash and chickpeas with warming spices and a hint of sourdough discard to add depth and a slight tang to this vibrant soup.

- **Recipe 87: Creamy Asparagus & Spinach Soup** A lush green soup that combines the freshness of asparagus and spinach with a creamy base, where sourdough discard adds a hint of complexity and enriches the texture.

- **Recipe 88: Classic Gazpacho**: Revitalized Refresh with a cold serving of this classic Spanish soup, revitalized with a blend of fresh vegetables and sourdough bread infused with vinegar and olive oil, making it a perfect summer refreshment.

Through these recipes, "Soups & Stews to Pair with Sourdough" not only offers a guide to making delicious meals but also teaches how to integrate sourdough in creative ways to elevate the culinary experience. Enjoy these soups and stews as they bring warmth and satisfaction to your table, proving that sourdough is indeed a baker's delight that goes well beyond the breadbasket.

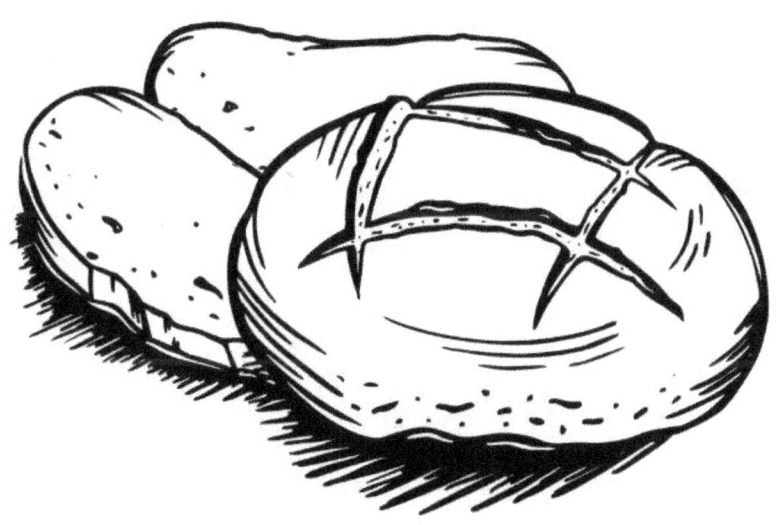

Adjust Hydration Based on Flour: "Different flours absorb water differently. Start with the recipe's recommended hydration level and adjust based on the dough's feel. A properly hydrated dough should be tacky but not excessively sticky."

Recipe 83: Creamy Carrot & Quinoa Soup

Prep Time: 15 mins | **Cook Time:** 30-35 mins | **Servings:** 4-6

Ingredients:

- 1 tablespoon olive oil
- 1/2 cup chopped onion.
- 4-5 medium carrots peeled and chopped.
- 1/2 cup cooked quinoa
- 4 cups vegetable broth
- 1/4 cup sourdough discard (brown rice or sorghum starter is preferable)
- 1/2 teaspoon dried thyme (or 1 teaspoon fresh)
- Salt and pepper to taste
- Optional: 1/4 cup heavy cream or cashew cream

Best Sourdough Starter: A mild, neutral starter complements the delicate carrot and quinoa flavors.

Step-by-Step Instructions:

1. **Sauté:** Sauté onions in olive oil until softened. Add carrots and cook for a few minutes more.
2. **Simmer:** Add quinoa, vegetable broth, thyme, sourdough discard, salt, and pepper. Bring to a boil, then reduce heat and simmer for 20-25 minutes or until carrots are tender.
3. **Blend:** Using an immersion blender (or in batches in a regular blender), puree the soup until smooth and creamy.
4. **Optional Creamy Finish:** If desired, stir in heavy cream or cashew cream for extra richness.
5. **Serve:** Taste and adjust seasoning. Garnish with fresh herbs if desired.

Nutritional Values (per 1 cup serving):

- Calories: 180
- Carbohydrates: 25g
- Protein: 8g
- Fat: 7g
- Sodium: 350mg
- Fiber: 5g

Cooking Tips:

- Add a pinch of curry powder or other spices for extra flavor depth.
- Top with a drizzle of olive oil, a dollop of yogurt, or a sprinkle of toasted nuts for extra richness.

Special Diets:

- **Vegetarian**: This recipe is already vegetarian-friendly!
- **Vegan**: Use a plant-based cream alternative or omit the cream entirely.
- **Gluten-free:** Ensure your vegetable broth is gluten-free.

Recipe 84: Hearty Lentil & Kale Stew

Prep Time: 15 mins | **Cook Time:** 30-35 mins | **Servings:** 4-6

Ingredients:

- 1 tablespoon olive oil
- 1/2 cup chopped onion.
- 2 cloves garlic, minced.
- 1 cup dried green or brown lentils, rinsed.
- 4 cups vegetable broth
- 1 can (14 oz) diced tomatoes.
- 1/4 cup sourdough discard (any variety)
- 1 teaspoon dried thyme
- 1 teaspoon dried oregano
- 4 cups chopped kale.
- Salt and pepper to taste

Best Sourdough Starter: Any starter will work – the lentils and kale offer dominant flavors.

Alternative Ingredients:

- Substitute dried lentils with other cooked lentils or beans.
- Use other leafy greens like spinach or Swiss chard instead of kale.

Step-by-Step Instructions:

1. **Sauté:** Sauté onions and garlic in olive oil until softened.
2. **Simmer:** Add lentils, vegetable broth, diced tomatoes, sourdough discard, thyme, oregano, salt, and pepper. Bring to a boil, then reduce heat and simmer for 25-30 minutes or until lentils are tender.
3. **Add Kale:** Stir in the chopped kale and cook for another 5 minutes or until the kale is wilted.
4. **Serve:** Taste and adjust seasoning. Serve with crusty sourdough bread for dipping.

Nutritional Values (per 1 cup serving):

- Calories: 200
- Carbohydrates: 30g
- Protein: 12g
- Fat: 5g
- Sodium: 300mg
- Fiber: 10g

Cooking Tips:

- ✓ Add a sprinkle of red pepper flakes for a touch of heat.
- ✓ Top with a sprinkle of parmesan cheese or nutritional yeast for a cheesy flavor.

Special Diets:

- **Vegan**: This recipe is already vegan-friendly!
- **Gluten-free**: Ensure your vegetable broth is gluten-free and serve with gluten-free bread.

Recipe 85: Tomato & White Bean Bisque

Prep Time: 15 mins | **Cook Time:** 35-40 mins (including roasting) | **Servings:** 4-6

Ingredients:

- 2-pounds of ripe tomatoes halved or quartered.
- 2 tablespoons olive oil
- 1/2 cup chopped onion.
- 2 cloves garlic, minced.
- 1 can (15oz) white beans, drained and rinsed.
- 4 cups vegetable broth
- 1/4 cup sourdough discard (any variety)
- 1/4 cup heavy cream or cashew cream
- 1 tablespoon dried basil
   Salt and pepper to taste

Best Sourdough Starter: Any starter will work – the roasted tomato and basil will be the dominant flavors.

Step-by-Step Instructions:

1. **Roast Tomatoes:** Toss tomatoes with a drizzle of olive oil, salt, and pepper. Roast in a preheated oven at 400°F (200°C) for 20-25 minutes or until slightly charred and softened.
2. **Sauté:** Sauté onions and garlic in remaining olive oil until softened.
3. **Simmer:** Add white beans, roasted tomatoes, vegetable broth, sourdough discard, heavy cream (or cashew cream), basil, salt, and pepper. Bring to a boil, then reduce heat and simmer for 10-15 minutes.
4. **Blend:** Using an immersion blender (or in batches in a regular blender), puree the soup until smooth and creamy.
5. **Serve:** Taste and adjust seasoning. Serve with a dollop of sour cream or yogurt and a sprinkle of fresh basil.

Nutritional Values (per 1 cup serving):

- Calories: 220
- Carbohydrates: 30g
- Protein: 10g
- Fat: 10g
- Sodium: 380mg
- Fiber: 8g

Cooking Tips:

- Use fire-roasted canned tomatoes for a shortcut and an extra smoky flavor.
- Garnish with a drizzle of pesto or balsamic glaze for an extra touch.

Special Diets:

- **Vegetarian**: This recipe is already vegetarian-friendly!
- **Vegan**: Use a plant-based cream alternative or omit the cream entirely.

Recipe 86: Spiced Butternut Squash & Chickpea Soup

Prep Time: 15 mins | **Cook Time:** 45-50 mins (including roasting) | **Servings:** 4-6

Ingredients:

- 1 medium butternut squash, peeled, seeded, and cubed.
- 2 tablespoons olive oil
- 1/2 cup chopped onion.
- 2 cloves garlic, minced.
- 1 can (15oz) chickpeas, drained and rinsed.
- 4 cups vegetable broth
- 1/4 cup coconut milk
- 1 tablespoon grated ginger
- 1 teaspoon ground cinnamon
- 1/2 teaspoon ground turmeric
- 1/4 cup sourdough discard (any variety)
- Salt and pepper to taste

Best Sourdough Starter: Any starter will work – the squash and spices provide the most flavor impact.

Step-by-Step Instructions:

1. **Roast Squash:** Toss squash cubes with a drizzle of olive oil, salt, and pepper. Roast in a preheated oven at 400°F (200°C) for 25-30 minutes or until tender and slightly caramelized.
2. **Sauté:** Sauté onions and garlic in remaining olive oil until softened.
3. **Simmer:** Add chickpeas, roasted squash, vegetable broth, coconut milk, ginger, cinnamon, turmeric, sourdough discard, salt, and pepper. Bring to a boil, then reduce heat and simmer for 15-20 minutes.
4. **Blend:** Using an immersion blender (or in batches in a regular blender), puree the soup until smooth and creamy.
5. **Serve:** Taste and adjust seasoning. Serve with a dollop of yogurt or a swirl of coconut cream.

Nutritional Values (per 1 cup serving):

- Calories: 250
- Carbohydrates: 35g
- Protein: 10g
- Fat: 12g
- Sodium: 350mg
- Fiber: 10g

Cooking Tips:

- Add a pinch of cayenne pepper for a touch of heat.
- Garnish with fresh cilantro or parsley and toasted pumpkin seeds for extra flavor and texture.

Special Diets:

- **Vegan**: This recipe is already vegan-friendly!
- **Gluten-free:** Ensure your vegetable broth is gluten-free.

Recipe 87: Creamy Asparagus & Spinach Soup

Prep Time: 15 mins | **Cook Time:** 20-25 mins | **Servings:** 4-6

Ingredients:

- 1 pound asparagus, tough ends trimmed and cut into pieces.
- 1 tablespoon olive oil
- 1/2 cup chopped onion.
- 1 medium potato peeled and diced.
- 4 cups vegetable broth
- 5 ounces baby spinach
- 1/4 cup heavy cream or cashew cream
- 1/4 cup sourdough discard (any variety)
- 1 teaspoon lemon zest
- Pinch of ground nutmeg
- Salt and pepper to taste

Best Sourdough Starter: Any starter will work – the asparagus and spinach provide the most flavor impact.

Step-by-Step Instructions:

1. **Sauté:** Sauté onions in olive oil until softened. Add asparagus and potato and cook for a few minutes more.
2. **Simmer:** Add vegetable broth and sourdough, and discard salt and pepper. Bring to a boil, then reduce heat and simmer for 15-20 minutes, or until asparagus and potato are tender.
3. **Add spinach:** Stir in spinach and cook until wilted for about 2 minutes.
4. **Blend:** Using an immersion blender (or in batches in a regular blender), puree the soup until smooth and creamy. Stir in cream, lemon zest, and nutmeg.
5. **Serve:** Taste and adjust seasoning. Serve hot, garnished with a dollop of sour cream or a sprinkle of toasted pine nuts, if desired.

Nutritional Values (per 1 cup serving):

- ❖ Calories: 150
- ❖ Carbohydrates: 20g
- ❖ Protein: 6g
- ❖ Fat: 7g
- ❖ Sodium: 320mg
- ❖ Fiber: 5g

Cooking Tips:

- ✓ Use frozen chopped spinach for convenience.
- ✓ Add a handful of fresh herbs like basil or parsley for extra flavor.

Special Diets:

- **Vegetarian**: This recipe is already vegetarian-friendly!
- **Vegan**: Use a plant-based cream alternative or omit the cream entirely.

Recipe 88: Classic Gazpacho: Revitalized

Prep Time: 15 mins + chilling time | **Cook Time:** None | **Servings:** 4-6

Ingredients:

- 2 pounds ripe tomatoes roughly chopped.
- 1 cucumber, peeled, seeded, and chopped.
- 1 green bell pepper seeded and chopped.
- 1/2 cup chopped onion.
- 2 cloves garlic, minced.
- 1/2 cup crusty sourdough bread, soaked in water and squeezed dry.
- 1/4 cup olive oil
- 2 tablespoons sherry vinegar (or red wine vinegar)
- 1/4 cup sourdough discard (any variety)
- Salt and pepper to taste

Best Sourdough Starter: A tangy starter would complement the bright flavors of the gazpacho nicely.

Step-by-Step Instructions:

1. **Soak Bread:** Soak the crusty sourdough bread in a small amount of water for a few minutes, then squeeze out excess liquid.
2. **Blend:** Combine tomatoes, cucumber, bell pepper, onion, garlic, soaked bread, olive oil, sherry vinegar, sourdough discard, salt, and pepper in a blender. Blend until smooth or to your desired consistency (slightly chunky is traditional).
3. **Chill:** Refrigerate for at least 2 hours, or preferably overnight, to allow flavors to meld.
4. **Serve:** Taste and adjust the seasoning before serving. Garnish with chopped fresh herbs, a drizzle of olive oil, or croutons.

Nutritional Values (per 1 cup serving):

- ❖ Calories: 150
- ❖ Carbohydrates: 20g
- ❖ Protein: 4g
- ❖ Fat: 8g
- ❖ Sodium: 300mg
- ❖ Fiber: 4g

Cooking Tips:

- ✓ For an extra smooth gazpacho, strain the soup after blending and before chilling.
- ✓ Experiment with different garnishes like diced avocado, crumbled feta cheese, or chopped fresh basil.

Special Diets:

- **Vegan:** This recipe is already vegan-friendly!
- **Gluten-free:** Ensure you use gluten-free bread.

Chapter 20: Salad Dressings Enhanced by Sourdough Crumbs (6 Recipes)

In this unique and exploratory chapter of our culinary collection, "Salad Dressings Enhanced by Sourdough Crumbs," we dive into the delightful world of salads but with a twist that transforms the ordinary into the extraordinary. Salad dressings are an integral part of any salad, often defining the flavor and character of the dish. However, when you introduce the rustic, earthy flavors of sourdough crumbs, you elevate these dressings to a new level of texture and taste.

As you venture through these six innovative recipes, you'll discover how the humble sourdough breadcrumb can add not only crunch and depth to your dressings but also a way to utilize leftover bread that might otherwise be discarded. This chapter is designed not just to inspire your taste buds but also to encourage a more sustainable approach to cooking.

Each recipe in this chapter has been carefully crafted to showcase how sourdough crumbs, whether fresh or toasted, can enhance the natural flavors of traditional and modern salad dressings. From creamy concoctions to tangy vinaigrettes, these dressings are versatile. They can be used to dress leafy greens, drizzle over grilled vegetables, or even marinate proteins. The inclusion of sourdough crumbs adds a pleasing texture and a slight nuttiness that complements various salad components beautifully.

Why Sourdough Crumbs?

Sourdough bread, known for its distinct tang and chewy texture, makes for crumbs that are not just filler but a feature that offers both flavor and function. These crumbs absorb and meld the flavors of the dressing ingredients more harmoniously than their fresher, softer counterparts, providing an extended flavor profile that develops as the dressing sits.

Exploring the Recipes

Each recipe in this chapter will guide you through the process of creating dressings that are both nutritious and delicious, ensuring that every salad is as pleasing to the palate as it is to the eye. We will explore a variety of flavors, from a rich and creamy blue cheese dressing sprinkled with sourdough crumbs to a zesty citrus vinaigrette that uses the crumbs to thicken and enhance the dressing's body.

Moreover, this chapter isn't just about following recipes—it's about inspiring you to experiment with textures and flavors. You'll learn how to balance the acidity of the dressings with the subtle sourness of the sourdough and how different seasoning techniques can alter the profile of the crumbs from mildly toasted to deeply caramelized.

What You Will Gain

By the end of this chapter, you'll have not only expanded your repertoire of salad dressings but also gained a deeper appreciation for the versatility of sourdough bread beyond the usual applications. Whether you're a seasoned chef or a home cook looking to bring new life to your salads, these recipes offer a gateway to enhancing your culinary skills and enriching your dining experience.

Join us on this flavorful journey as we blend, mix, and toss our way through the art of salad dressing creation, proving once and for all that even the smallest ingredient, like a breadcrumb, can make a world of difference in the craft of cooking.

Recipes:

Recipe 89: Creamy Herb & Sourdough Crumb Vinaigrette: Combine sourdough breadcrumbs, olive oil, white wine vinegar, Dijon mustard, fresh herbs, garlic, and a touch of honey.

Recipe 90: Roasted Garlic & Parmesan Vinaigrette: Toast sourdough breadcrumbs with roasted garlic and grated parmesan. Mix with olive oil, balsamic vinegar, and a sprinkle of dried oregano.

Recipe 91: Tahini, Lemon & Sourdough Crumb Dressing: Blend sourdough breadcrumbs, tahini, lemon juice, olive oil, water, a hint of garlic, and a pinch of cumin for a creamy and vibrant dressing.

Recipe 92: Spiced Carrot & Ginger Dressing: Grate carrots, blend with sourdough breadcrumbs, ginger, olive oil, rice vinegar, a dash of soy sauce, and a sprinkle of sesame seeds.

Recipe 93: Avocado & Lime Vinaigrette: Blend avocado, sourdough breadcrumbs, lime juice, olive oil, cilantro, a hint of jalapeño, and a touch of honey.

Recipe 94: Balsamic & Berry Vinaigrette: Muddle berries (raspberries, blueberries), then whisk with balsamic vinegar, olive oil, sourdough breadcrumbs, herbs, and a touch of Dijon mustard.

Recipe 89: Creamy Herb & Sourdough Crumb Vinaigrette

Prep Time: 10 mins | **Yield:** About 1 cup

Ingredients:

- 1/2 cup sourdough breadcrumbs
- 1/4 cup olive oil
- 2 tablespoons white wine vinegar (or red wine vinegar)
- 1 tablespoon Dijon mustard
- 2 tablespoons chopped fresh herbs (parsley, basil, chives, etc.)
- 1 clove garlic, minced.
- 1/2 teaspoon honey
- Salt and pepper to taste

Step-by-Step Instructions:

1. **Toast Breadcrumbs (optional):** For a deeper flavor, lightly toast the breadcrumbs in a dry skillet over medium heat until golden brown.
2. **Combine:** In a jar or bowl, combine breadcrumbs, olive oil, vinegar, mustard, herbs, garlic, honey, salt, and pepper.
3. **Shake or Whisk:** Seal the jar tightly and shake vigorously or whisk in a bowl until well emulsified.
4. **Taste & Serve:** Adjust seasoning with salt, pepper, or additional honey to your liking. Use immediately or store in the refrigerator.

Serving Suggestions:

- Drizzle over leafy green salads with fresh vegetables.
- Use as a marinade for grilled chicken or fish.
- Toss with roasted vegetables for extra flavor.

Nutritional Values (per 2 tablespoons):

- Calories: 100
- Carbohydrates: 5g
- Protein: 2g
- Fat: 9g
- Sodium: 100mg
- Fiber: 1g

Cooking Tips:

- Experiment with different herb combinations.
- Add a touch of lemon zest for a citrusy brightness.

Special Diets:

- **Vegetarian**: This recipe is already vegetarian-friendly!
- **Vegan**: Substitute the honey with maple syrup. Ensure your mustard is vegan-friendly.

Recipe 90: Roasted Garlic & Parmesan Vinaigrette

Prep Time: 15 mins (+ garlic roasting time) | **Cook Time:** 30-40 mins (roasting) | **Yield:** About 1 cup

Ingredients:

- 1 head of garlic
- 1/2 cup sourdough breadcrumbs
- 1/4 cup grated parmesan cheese.
- 1/4 cup olive oil
- 2 tablespoons balsamic vinegar
- 1 teaspoon dried oregano (or other Italian herbs)
- Salt and pepper to taste

Best Sourdough Starter: A mild, neutral starter complements the roasted garlic and parmesan flavors.

Step-by-Step Instructions:

1. **Roast Garlic:** Cut the top off a head of garlic, drizzle with olive oil, wrap in foil, and roast in a preheated oven at 400°F (200°C) for 30-40 minutes or until soft and caramelized.
2. **Toast Breadcrumbs:** Lightly toast the breadcrumbs in a dry skillet over medium heat until golden brown.
3. **Combine:** Squeeze the roasted garlic cloves out of their skins. In a jar or bowl, combine breadcrumbs, roasted garlic, parmesan cheese, olive oil, balsamic vinegar, oregano, salt, and pepper.
4. **Shake or Whisk:** Seal the jar tightly and shake vigorously or whisk in a bowl until well emulsified.
5. **Taste & Serve:** Adjust seasoning with salt, pepper, or additional balsamic vinegar to your liking. Use immediately or store in the refrigerator.

Serving Suggestions:

- Dress a classic Italian salad with tomatoes, cucumbers, and olives.
- Drizzle over grilled vegetables or roasted potatoes.
- Use as a dipping sauce for breadsticks or crusty bread.

Nutritional Values (per 2 tablespoons):

- Calories: 120
- Carbohydrates: 5g
- Protein: 4g
- Fat: 10g
- Sodium: 150mg
- Fiber: 1g

Cooking Tips:

- ✓ Use pre-roasted garlic from a jar for a time-saving shortcut.
- ✓ Add a pinch of red pepper flakes for a touch of heat.

Special Diets:

- **Vegetarian**: This recipe is already vegetarian-friendly!
- **Vegan**: Substitute the parmesan cheese with a vegan alternative or nutritional yeast.

Recipe 91: Tahini, Lemon & Sourdough Crumb Dressing

Prep Time: 10 mins | **Yield:** About 1 cup

Ingredients:

- 1/2 cup sourdough breadcrumbs
- 1/4 cup tahini
- 1/4 cup lemon juice
- 1/4 cup olive oil
- 2-3 tablespoons water (more as needed)
- 1 clove garlic, minced.
- 1/4 teaspoon ground cumin
- Salt and pepper to taste

Best Sourdough Starter: Any starter will work – the tahini and lemon provide the dominant flavors.

Alternative Ingredients:

- Substitute tahini with other nuts or seed butter like sunflower seed butter or almond butter.

Step-by-Step Instructions:

1. **Combine:** In a blender or food processor, combine breadcrumbs, tahini, lemon juice, olive oil, water, garlic, cumin, salt, and pepper.
2. **Blend & Thin:** Blend until smooth, adding more water as needed to achieve desired consistency.
3. **Taste & Serve:** Adjust seasoning with salt, pepper, or additional lemon juice to your liking. Use immediately or store in the refrigerator.

Serving Suggestions:

- Drizzle over salads with chickpeas, cucumbers, tomatoes, and feta cheese.
- Use as a dip for pita bread or raw vegetables.
- Toss with roasted cauliflower or other vegetables.

Nutritional Values (per 2 tablespoons):

- Calories: 130
- Carbohydrates: 5g
- Protein: 4g
- Fat: 11g
- Sodium: 100mg
- Fiber: 1g

Cooking Tips:

- Add a pinch of cayenne pepper for a touch of heat.
- Garnish with chopped fresh parsley or cilantro for a pop of color.

Special Diets:

- **Vegan**: This recipe is already vegan-friendly!
- **Gluten-free:** Ensure you use gluten-free breadcrumbs.

Recipe 92: Spiced Carrot & Ginger Dressing

Prep Time: 10 mins | **Yield:** About 1 cup

Ingredients:

- 1/2 cup grated carrots.
- 1/4 cup sourdough breadcrumbs
- 1 tablespoon grated fresh ginger.
- 1/4 cup olive oil
- 2 tablespoons rice vinegar
- 1 teaspoon soy sauce
- 1 teaspoon sesame oil
- Pinch of red pepper flakes (optional)
- Salt and pepper to taste

Best Sourdough Starter: Any starter will work; the carrot and ginger provide the dominant flavor notes.

Step-by-Step Instructions:

1. **Combine:** In a blender or food processor, combine grated carrots, breadcrumbs, ginger, olive oil, rice vinegar, soy sauce, sesame oil, red pepper flakes (if using), salt, and pepper.
2. **Blend:** Blend until mostly smooth, with some small pieces of carrot for texture.
3. **Taste & Serve:** Adjust seasoning with salt, pepper, or additional rice vinegar to your liking. Use immediately or store in the refrigerator.

Serving Suggestions:

- Dress a salad with Asian-inspired ingredients like Napa cabbage, edamame, and mandarin oranges.
- Use as a dipping sauce for spring rolls or dumplings.
- Drizzle over grilled chicken or tofu for a flavorful boost.

Nutritional Values (per 2 tablespoons):

- Calories: 110
- Carbohydrates: 7g
- Protein: 2g
- Fat: 9g
- Sodium: 180mg
- Fiber: 2g

Cooking Tips:

- Add a sprinkle of toasted sesame seeds for a nutty garnish.
- Substitute rice vinegar with white wine vinegar or apple cider vinegar.

Special Diets:

- **Vegetarian:** This recipe is already vegetarian-friendly!
- **Vegan:** Ensure your soy sauce is vegan-friendly.
- **Gluten-free:** Ensure you use gluten-free breadcrumbs.

Recipe 93: Avocado & Lime Vinaigrette

Prep Time: 10 mins | **Yield:** About 1 cup

Ingredients:

- 1/2 ripe avocado peeled and pitted.
- 1/4 cup sourdough breadcrumbs
- 1/4 cup lime juice
- 1/4 cup olive oil
- 2 tablespoons chopped cilantro.
- 1/2 jalapeño pepper, seeded and finely diced (optional)
- 1/2 teaspoon honey (or maple syrup)
- Salt and pepper to taste

Best Sourdough Starter: Any starter will work – the avocado and lime are the stars here.

Alternative Ingredients:

- Substitute jalapeño pepper with a milder pepper like Anaheim or remove it for a non-spicy version.

Step-by-Step Instructions:

1. **Combine:** In a blender or food processor, combine avocado, breadcrumbs, lime juice, olive oil, cilantro, jalapeño (if using), honey, salt, and pepper.
2. **Blend:** Blend until smooth and creamy.
3. **Taste & Serve:** Adjust seasoning with salt, pepper, or additional lime juice to your liking. Use immediately or store in the refrigerator.

Serving Suggestions:

- Drizzle over a salad with black beans, corn, tomatoes, and bell peppers for a Southwest-inspired flavor.
- Use as a dip for quesadillas or tacos.
- Toss with grilled shrimp or fish for a light and refreshing meal.

Nutritional Values (per 2 tablespoons):

- Calories: 120
- Carbohydrates: 5g
- Protein: 2g
- Fat: 11g
- Sodium: 80mg
- Fiber: 2g

Cooking Tips:

- For a spicier dressing, leave some seeds in the jalapeño pepper.
- Add a touch of cumin or smoked paprika for a more complex flavor profile.

Special Diets:

- **Vegetarian**: This recipe is already vegetarian-friendly!
- **Vegan**: Ensure your honey is replaced with maple syrup or another plant-based sweetener.
- **Gluten-free:** Ensure you use gluten-free breadcrumbs.

Recipe 94: Balsamic & Berry Vinaigrette

Prep Time: 10 mins | **Yield:** About 1 cup

Ingredients:

- 1/2 cup fresh berries (raspberries, blueberries, or a mix)
- 1/4 cup sourdough breadcrumbs
- 1/4 cup balsamic vinegar
- 1/4 cup olive oil
- 1 teaspoon Dijon mustard
- 1 tablespoon chopped fresh herbs (basil, thyme, or mint)
- Salt and pepper to taste

Best Sourdough Starter: Any starter will work – the berries and balsamic vinegar provide the dominant flavors.

Alternative Ingredients:

- Use frozen berries that have been thawed and drained of excess liquid.
- Substitute balsamic vinegar with red wine vinegar or apple cider vinegar.

Step-by-Step Instructions:

1. **Muddle Berries:** In a small bowl, muddle the berries gently to release some of their juices.
2. **Combine:** In a jar or bowl, whisk together the muddled berries, breadcrumbs, balsamic vinegar, olive oil, Dijon mustard, herbs, salt, and pepper.
3. **Shake or Whisk:** Seal the jar tightly and shake vigorously or whisk in a bowl until well emulsified.
4. **Taste & Serve:** Adjust seasoning with salt, pepper, or additional balsamic vinegar to your liking. Use immediately or store in the refrigerator.

Serving Suggestions:

- Dress a salad with spinach, goat cheese, and toasted walnuts for a classic combination.
- Drizzle over grilled chicken or salmon for a sweet and tangy flavor boost.
- Use as a dip for fresh fruit or crusty bread.

Nutritional Values (per 2 tablespoons):

- ❖ Calories: 100
- ❖ Carbohydrates: 6g
- ❖ Protein: 2g
- ❖ Fat: 9g
- ❖ Sodium: 80mg
- ❖ Fiber: 2g

Cooking Tips:

- ✓ Let the vinaigrette sit for a few minutes before serving to allow the flavors to meld.
- ✓ Add a touch of maple syrup or honey for extra sweetness.

Special Diets:

- **Vegetarian**: This recipe is already vegetarian-friendly!
- **Vegan**: Ensure your Dijon mustard is vegan-friendly.
- **Gluten-free**: Ensure you use gluten-free breadcrumbs.

Chapter 21: Creative Sourdough Crumb Uses (7 Recipes)

Welcome to Chapter 21, "Creative Sourdough Crumb Uses," where we explore innovative and delicious ways to repurpose leftover sourdough crumbs. This chapter is dedicated to sustainability and creativity, showing you how to transform what might otherwise be wasted into culinary treasures. Through seven unique recipes, we'll dive into the versatility of sourdough crumbs, turning them into flavorful additions to both savory and sweet dishes.

Sourdough crumbs, often overlooked, hold immense potential for enhancing texture and flavor. They can be used as a crunchy topping for casseroles, a binder for meatballs, or even as a base for delectable dessert crusts. This chapter will guide you through various techniques to incorporate these flavorful bits into your cooking, elevating everyday meals into something extraordinary.

Here's what you'll find in this chapter:
Recipes that range from simple garnishes to main components, showing the full scope of what sourdough crumbs can do.

Tips on how to properly dry and store sourdough crumbs for maximum flavor and usability.
Ideas for seasoning and enhancing sourdough crumbs to suit any type of dish.

Embrace the art of zero-waste baking as you learn to see sourdough crumbs not as leftovers, but as ingredients full of possibility. Let's get creative and make the most out of every bit of sourdough!

Recipe 95: Herb-Crusted Fish: Coat fish fillets in a mixture of sourdough breadcrumbs, herbs, and a hint of lemon zest. Bake or pan-fry for a crispy, flavorful crust.

Recipe 96: Quinoa & Sourdough Stuffed Peppers: Combine cooked quinoa, ground turkey, diced vegetables, marinara sauce, and sourdough breadcrumbs for a hearty filling.

Recipe 97: Roasted Vegetable Gratin: Top layered roasted vegetables (zucchini, eggplant, tomatoes) with a blend of sourdough crumbs, parmesan, herbs, and a drizzle of olive oil.

Recipe 98: Roasted Cauliflower Steaks: Coat cauliflower steaks in sourdough crumbs spiced with paprika and cumin, then roast until golden brown.

Recipe 99: Baked Mac & Cheese Topping: A decadent mix of sourdough breadcrumbs, butter, and parmesan for a crisp and flavorful topping on your favorite mac & cheese.

Recipe 100: Savory Breakfast Crumble: Sauté spinach, mushrooms, and onions. Top with eggs and a sprinkle of sourdough breadcrumbs mixed with feta cheese. Bake until set.

Recipe 101: Fruit & Sourdough Crumble: Combine chopped fruit (apples, berries) with a topping of sourdough breadcrumbs, oats, nuts, brown sugar, and spices. Bake for a warm, bubbly dessert.

Recipe 95: Herb-Crusted Fish

Prep Time: 10 mins | **Cook Time:** Varies depending on the type of fish

Ingredients:

- 1 cup sourdough breadcrumbs
- 1/4 cup chopped fresh herbs (parsley, thyme, basil, etc.)
- 1 tablespoon lemon zest
- 1/4 teaspoon salt
- 1/4 teaspoon black pepper
- 4 (6-ounce) fish fillets (cod, halibut, tilapia, etc.)
- 1 tablespoon olive oil

Best Sourdough Starter: A mild, neutral starter complements the delicate fish flavors and fresh herbs.

Step-by-Step Instructions:

1. **Combine Crumb Mixture:** In a shallow bowl, combine sourdough breadcrumbs, herbs, lemon zest, salt, and pepper.
2. **Coat Fish:** Pat fish fillets dry with paper towels. Lightly brush with olive oil, then coat both sides with the crumb mixture, pressing gently to adhere.
3. **Cook:** Choose your preferred cooking method:
4. **Bake:** Preheat oven to 400°F (200°C). Bake fish on a lightly oiled baking sheet for 12-15 minutes or until cooked through.
5. **Pan-fry:** Heat a drizzle of olive oil in a skillet over medium heat. Cook fish for 3-4 minutes per side or until golden brown and cooked through.

Serving Suggestions:

- Serve with a squeeze of lemon and a side of steamed vegetables or a green salad.

Nutritional Values (per serving, assuming cod):

- ❖ Calories: 250
- ❖ Carbohydrates: 10g
- ❖ Protein: 30g
- ❖ Fat: 10g
- ❖ Sodium: 300mg
- ❖ Fiber: 2g

Cooking Tips:

- ✓ Adjust the herbs to your preference.
- ✓ Add a pinch of garlic powder or onion powder to the crumb mixture for extra flavor.

Special Diets:

- **Gluten-free:** Ensure you use gluten-free breadcrumbs.

Recipe 96: Quinoa & Sourdough Stuffed Peppers

Prep Time: 15 mins | **Cook Time:** 30-40 mins (includes quinoa cooking)

Ingredients:

- 1/2 cup quinoa, rinsed.
- 4 large bell peppers (any color)
- 1 tablespoon olive oil
- 1/2 cup chopped onion.
- 1 cup chopped vegetables (zucchini, mushrooms, carrots, etc.)
- 1 can (15oz) diced tomatoes, undrained.
- 1/2 cup cooked ground turkey (or other ground meat)
- 1/2 cup sourdough breadcrumbs
- 1/2 cup marinara sauce
- 1/2 cup shredded mozzarella cheese (optional)
- Salt and pepper to taste

Best Sourdough Starter: Any starter will work – the filling has a variety of flavors that will be dominant.

Alternative Ingredients:

- Substitute quinoa with cooked rice, lentils, or other grains.
- Use your favorite type of ground meat, or substitute with crumbled tofu for a vegetarian option.

Step-by-Step Instructions:

1. **Cook Quinoa:** Cook quinoa according to package directions.
2. **Prep Peppers:** Cut tops off bell peppers and remove seeds.
3. **Sauté:** Heat olive oil in a skillet. Sauté onion and vegetables until softened.
4. **Make Filling:** Add diced tomatoes, ground turkey (or substitute), cooked quinoa, breadcrumbs, marinara sauce, salt, and pepper to the skillet. Cook for a few minutes to combine flavors.
5. **Stuff Peppers:** Fill the hollowed-out bell peppers with the quinoa mixture.
6. **Bake:** Place stuffed peppers in a baking dish. Bake in a preheated oven at 375°F (190°C) for 30-40 minutes, or until peppers are tender and filling is heated through. Top with cheese (if using) during the last few minutes of baking.

Nutritional Values (per stuffed pepper):

- ❖ Calories: 350
- ❖ Carbohydrates: 35g
- ❖ Protein: 25g
- ❖ Fat: 15g
- ❖ Sodium: 450mg
- ❖ Fiber: 6g

Cooking Tips:

- ✓ Add a sprinkle of your favorite spices to the filling for extra flavor.
- ✓ If you don't have marinara sauce, use tomato sauce and a pinch of Italian seasoning.

Special Diets:

- **Gluten-free**: Ensure you use gluten-free breadcrumbs.

Recipe 97: Roasted Vegetable Gratin

Prep Time: 20 mins | **Cook Time:** 35-45 mins

Ingredients:

- 2-3 medium zucchini, sliced.
- 1 medium eggplant, sliced.
- 2 large tomatoes, sliced.
- 1 tablespoon olive oil
- 1/2 cup sourdough breadcrumbs
- 1/4 cup grated parmesan cheese.
- 2 tablespoons chopped fresh herbs (basil, oregano, thyme, etc.)
- 1 tablespoon olive oil, extra
- Salt and pepper to taste

Best Sourdough Starter: Any starter will work – the roasted vegetables and herbs provide the dominant flavors.

Alternative Ingredients:

- Feel free to use other seasonal vegetables like bell peppers, onions, or summer squash.

Step-by-Step Instructions:

1. **Roast Vegetables:** Preheat oven to 425°F (220°C). Toss sliced zucchini, eggplant, and tomatoes with olive oil, salt, and pepper. Spread out on a baking sheet and roast for 20-25 minutes or until tender and slightly browned.
2. **Make Topping:** While the vegetables roast, combine sourdough breadcrumbs, parmesan cheese, herbs, a drizzle of olive oil, salt, and pepper in a bowl.
3. **Assemble Gratin:** Arrange the roasted vegetables in a baking dish, overlapping slightly. Sprinkle the breadcrumbs topping evenly over the vegetables.
4. **Bake:** Bake for 15-20 minutes or until the topping is golden brown and bubbly.

Nutritional Values (per serving):

- Calories: 200
- Carbohydrates: 20g
- Protein: 8g
- Fat: 12g
- Sodium: 350mg
- Fiber: 6g

Cooking Tips:

- Cut the vegetables into uniform slices for even cooking.
- If you don't have fresh herbs, substitute with a teaspoon or two of dried Italian seasoning.

Special Diets:

- **Vegetarian**: This recipe is already vegetarian-friendly!
- **Gluten-free:** Ensure you use gluten-free breadcrumbs.

Recipe 98: Roasted Cauliflower Steaks

Prep Time: 15 mins | **Cook Time:** 25-30 mins

Ingredients:

- 1 large head of cauliflower
- 1/4 cup olive oil
- 1/2 cup sourdough breadcrumbs
- 1 teaspoon smoked paprika.
- 1/2 teaspoon cumin powder
- 1/4 teaspoon garlic powder
- Salt and pepper to taste

Best Sourdough Starter: A mild, neutral starter complements the smoky paprika and other spices.

Step-by-Step Instructions:

1. **Cut "Steaks":** Cut the cauliflower head into thick slices (about 1-inch thick) to create "steaks."
2. **Make Coating:** In a shallow bowl, combine olive oil, breadcrumbs, paprika, cumin, garlic powder, salt, and pepper.
3. **Coat Cauliflower:** Dip each cauliflower steak into the coating mixture, pressing gently to adhere.
4. **Roast:** Place coated cauliflower steaks on a baking sheet. Roast in a preheated oven at 425°F (220°C) for 20-25 minutes or until golden brown and tender.

Serving Suggestions:

- Serve as a vegetarian main dish with a side of roasted vegetables or a green salad.
- Top with a dollop of yogurt and a sprinkle of fresh herbs for a tangy twist.
- Drizzle with a creamy tahini sauce for extra richness.

Nutritional Values (per serving):

- Calories: 180
- Carbohydrates: 15g
- Protein: 6g
- Fat: 13g
- Sodium: 200mg
- Fiber: 5g

Cooking Tips:

- Add a pinch of cayenne pepper for a touch of heat.
- Experiment with different spice combinations to suit your taste.

Special Diets:

- **Vegetarian**: This recipe is already vegetarian-friendly!
- **Vegan**: This recipe is also vegan-friendly.
- **Gluten-free:** Ensure you use gluten-free breadcrumbs.

Recipe 99: Baked Mac & Cheese Topping

Prep Time: 5 mins | **Cook Time:** Varies depending on your mac & cheese recipe

Ingredients:

- 1/2 cup sourdough breadcrumbs
- 2 tablespoons melted butter.
- 1/4 cup grated parmesan cheese.
- Your favorite prepared mac & cheese

Best Sourdough Starter: Any starter will work – the butter and parmesan provide the majority of the flavor.

Step-by-Step Instructions:

1. **Make Topping:** In a bowl, combine sourdough breadcrumbs, melted butter, and parmesan cheese. Mix until well combined.
2. **Prepare Mac & Cheese:** Prepare your favorite mac & cheese according to the recipe instructions.
3. **Top & Bake:** Spread the mac & cheese in a baking dish. Sprinkle the breadcrumbs topping evenly over the mac & cheese. Bake according to your mac & cheese recipe instructions or until the topping is golden brown and bubbly.

Serving Suggestions:

- Enjoy as a comforting and satisfying side dish or main course.

Nutritional Values (per serving, topping only):

- ❖ Calories: 100
- ❖ Carbohydrates: 10g
- ❖ Protein: 4g
- ❖ Fat: 7g
- ❖ Sodium: 180mg
- ❖ Fiber: 1g

Cooking Tips:

- ✓ If you like a crunchier topping, lightly toast the breadcrumbs before mixing them with butter and parmesan.
- ✓ Add a sprinkle of your favorite herbs or spices for extra flavor.

Special Diets:

- **Gluten-free:** Ensure you use gluten-free breadcrumbs.

Recipe 100: Savory Breakfast Crumble

Prep Time: 15 mins | **Cook Time:** 20-25 mins.

Ingredients:

- 1 tablespoon olive oil
- 1 cup chopped spinach.
- 1/2 cup chopped mushrooms.
- 1/4 cup chopped onion.
- 6 eggs
- 1/4 cup milk (or dairy-free alternative)
- 1/2 cup sourdough breadcrumbs
- 1/4 cup crumbled feta cheese
- Salt and pepper to taste

Best Sourdough Starter: Any starter will work – the spinach, mushrooms, and feta provide the dominant flavors.

Alternative Ingredients:

- Use other vegetables like chopped bell peppers, zucchini, or tomatoes.
- Substitute feta cheese with goat cheese or shredded cheddar cheese.

Step-by-Step Instructions:

1. **Sauté:** Heat olive oil in a skillet. Sauté spinach, mushrooms, and onion until softened. Season with salt and pepper.
2. **Whisk Eggs:** In a bowl, whisk together eggs, milk, salt, and pepper.
3. **Make Crumble:** In a separate bowl, combine sourdough breadcrumbs and feta cheese.
4. **Assemble:** Spread the sautéed vegetables in a greased baking dish. Pour the egg mixture over the vegetables. Sprinkle the breadcrumbs-feta mixture on top.
5. **Bake:** Bake in a preheated oven at 375°F (190°C) for 20-25 minutes, or until the eggs are set and the topping is golden brown.

Serving Suggestions:

- Serve warm with a side of hot sauce or salsa for an extra kick.

Nutritional Values (per serving):

- Calories: 250
- Carbohydrates: 15g
- Protein: 20g
- Fat: 15g
- Sodium: 400mg
- Fiber: 4g

Cooking Tips:

- Don't overcook the eggs. They'll continue to set slightly even after you remove them from the oven.
- Add a sprinkle of your favorite spices to the egg mixture for extra flavor.

Special Diets:

- **Vegetarian:** This recipe is already vegetarian-friendly!
- **Gluten-free:** Ensure you use gluten-free breadcrumbs.

Recipe 101 Fruit & Sourdough Crumble

Prep Time: 15 mins | **Cook Time:** 30-35 mins

Ingredients:

Filling:

- 4 cups chopped fruit (apples, berries, peaches, etc.)
- 1/4 cup sugar
- 1 tablespoon lemon juice
- 1/2 teaspoon ground cinnamon (or other spices to match your fruit)

Crumble Topping:

- 1/2 cup sourdough breadcrumbs
- 1/4 cup all-purpose flour (or gluten-free alternative)
- 1/4 cup rolled oats.
- 1/4 cup chopped nuts (optional)
- 1/4 cup brown sugar
- 1/4 teaspoon ground cinnamon
- 5 tablespoons cold unsalted butter, cut into small pieces.

Best Sourdough Starter: Any starter will work – the fruit and spices provide the dominant flavors.

Step-by-Step Instructions:

1. **Make Filling:** In a bowl, toss together fruit, sugar, lemon juice, and cinnamon. Spread into a greased baking dish.
2. **Make Crumble Topping:** In another bowl, combine sourdough breadcrumbs, flour, oats, nuts (if using), brown sugar, and cinnamon. Using your fingers or a pastry cutter, rub in the cold butter until the mixture resembles coarse crumbs.
3. **Assemble & Bake:** Sprinkle the crumble topping evenly over the fruit. Bake in a preheated oven at 375°F (190°C) for 30-35 minutes, or until the fruit is bubbly and the topping is golden brown.

Serving Suggestions:

- Serve warm with a scoop of vanilla ice cream or whipped cream for extra indulgence.

Nutritional Values (per serving):

- Calories: 300
- Carbohydrates: 50g
- Protein: 5g
- Fat: 15g
- Sodium: 100mg
- Fiber: 5g

Cooking Tips:

✓ Use a mix of fruits for added flavor and texture.
✓ Add a pinch of nutmeg or ginger to the crumble topping for extra warmth.

Special Diets:

- **Gluten-free:** Ensure you use gluten-free breadcrumbs, flour, and oats.

Chapter 22: Nutritional Notes and Recipe Adaptations

In Chapter 22, we delve into the nutritional aspects of sourdough baking and explore how to adapt recipes to meet specific dietary needs. This chapter provides valuable insights into the health benefits of sourdough and offers practical tips for customizing recipes, whether you're aiming to reduce sodium, cut calories, or incorporate more fiber-rich ingredients.

Here, you'll find:
- Detailed nutritional profiles for key sourdough ingredients.
- Guidelines for adjusting recipes to fit gluten-free, low-carb, or dairy-free diets.
- Tips on how to enhance the nutritional value of your sourdough creations without compromising flavor.

This chapter is essential for anyone looking to make healthier baking choices while enjoying the delicious and unique qualities of sourdough.

Detailed Nutritional Profiles for Key Sourdough Ingredients

In our journey through the world of sourdough, understanding the nutritional value of the ingredients we use is essential. This section provides comprehensive nutritional profiles for key sourdough ingredients, helping you make informed decisions about the components of your bread and their health benefits.

1. **Whole Wheat Flour**:
    - **Calories**: Higher in calories than refined flour but packed with nutrients.
    - **Fiber**: Rich in dietary fiber, promoting digestive health.
    - **Proteins**: Contains more protein than refined flours, aiding in muscle repair and growth.
    - **Minerals**: A good source of selenium, potassium, and magnesium.
2. **Rye Flour**:
    - **Calories**: Slightly lower in calories than wheat flour.
    - **Fiber**: Exceptionally high in fiber, especially soluble fiber that helps control blood sugar levels.
    - **Vitamins**: Rich in B-vitamins which are essential for metabolic health.
    - **Minerals**: High in iron and magnesium, crucial for energy production and overall health.
3. **Sourdough Starter**:
    - **Probiotics**: Natural fermentation introduces beneficial probiotics, which enhance gut health.
    - **Phytic Acid**: Fermentation reduces phytic acid, increasing mineral absorption.
    - **Enzymes**: Contains enzymes that break down gluten, making it easier to digest.
4. **Salt**:
    - **Minerals**: Provides essential minerals, primarily sodium, necessary for fluid balance and nerve function.
    - **Iodine**: Often iodized, contributing to thyroid health.

5. Water:
- **Hydration**: Essential for the hydration of flour and activation of gluten.
- **No Calories**: Adds no extra calories, making it ideal for managing dough consistency without affecting caloric intake.

These nutritional profiles not only guide you in selecting ingredients but also in understanding how each contributes to the healthfulness of your sourdough bread. By knowing these details, you can tailor your sourdough recipes to better fit your nutritional needs and preferences, ensuring every loaf you bake is as healthy as it is delicious.

Guidelines for Adjusting Recipes to Fit Gluten-Free, Low-Carb, or Dairy-Free Diets

Adapting sourdough recipes to accommodate specific dietary needs can seem challenging, but with the right guidelines, you can easily modify ingredients to fit gluten-free, low-carb, or dairy-free diets without sacrificing the quality or taste of your bread. Here's how you can adjust your sourdough recipes:

1. Gluten-Free Adjustments:
Flour Substitutions: Replace traditional wheat flour with a blend of gluten-free flour. A combination of rice flour, tapioca flour, and a binder like xanthan gum or psyllium husk can mimic the texture and structure of gluten.
Starter Modifications: Create a gluten-free sourdough starter using gluten-free flour and follow the same fermentation process as traditional starters.
Additional Ingredients: Sometimes, adding an egg or apple cider vinegar helps improve the structure and rise of gluten-free sourdough.

2. Low-Carb Adjustments:
Flour Choices: Use low-carb flour alternatives like almond flour, coconut flour, or flaxseed meal. These flours offer lower carbohydrate content and add a nutritious boost.
Reducing Sugar: Eliminate or substitute any added sugars with low-carb sweeteners such as stevia or erythritol.
Bulk and Binding: Since low-carb flours lack the binding properties of gluten, consider using more eggs or a small amount of xanthan gum to help bind the dough and enhance texture.

3. Dairy-Free Adjustments:
Milk Substitutes: Replace cow's milk with non-dairy alternatives such as almond milk, oat milk, or coconut milk. Choose unsweetened varieties to avoid adding extra sugar.
Butter Alternatives: Use plant-based butters or oils like coconut oil or olive oil as a substitute for butter.
Avoiding Hidden Dairy: Be mindful of hidden dairy ingredients in commercial additives or flavorings and opt for dairy-free versions.

General Tips for All Adaptations:

Experiment with Ratios: Finding the perfect substitute often requires experimentation. Start with small batches to test different combinations and ratios before finalizing your recipe.

Adjust Leavening Agents: Depending on your adjustments, you may need to tweak the amount of starter or leavening agents to achieve the desired texture and rise.

Hydration Levels: Different flours absorb water at different rates. Pay attention to the hydration level of your dough and adjust liquids as necessary to achieve a workable consistency.

By following these guidelines, you can tailor sourdough recipes to meet your dietary requirements while still enjoying the unique flavors and health benefits of sourdough bread. Whether you're avoiding gluten, reducing carbs, or cutting out dairy, these adjustments will help you bake delicious, inclusive sourdough bread that everyone can enjoy.

Tips on How to Enhance the Nutritional Value of Your Sourdough Creations Without Compromising Flavor

Enhancing the nutritional value of your sourdough creations is a rewarding endeavor that can yield delicious and healthful results. By incorporating a few thoughtful adjustments and additions, you can boost the nutritional profile of your sourdough breads while maintaining, or even enhancing, their flavor. Here are some tips to help you achieve this balance:

1. Incorporate Whole Grains:
- **Diverse Flours:** Substitute a portion of white flour with whole grain flour such as whole wheat, spelt, or rye. These flours not only increase the fiber content but also enrich the bread with vitamins and minerals.
- **Ancient Grains:** Add grains like quinoa, amaranth, or teff to your dough. These grains offer a spectrum of nutrients including protein, fiber, and essential amino acids.

2. Add Seeds and Nuts:
- **Nutrient Boost:** Mix seeds such as flaxseed, chia, sunflower, or pumpkin seeds into your dough. Nuts and seeds are excellent sources of healthy fats, proteins, and fiber.
- **Texture and Flavor:** Besides nutritional benefits, seeds and nuts also add a pleasant crunch and depth of flavor to your bread, enhancing its overall appeal.

3. Experiment with Sprouted Grains:
- **Enhanced Nutrition:** Sprouted grains have increased levels of vitamins and minerals, and decreased antinutrient levels, making nutrients more available for absorption.
- **Unique Flavor:** Sprouted grains can add a sweet and nutty flavor to bread, offering a delightful taste profile without the need for additional sugars.

4. Opt for Natural Sweeteners:
- **Healthier Options:** Reduce refined sugars by using alternatives like honey, maple syrup, or molasses, which also impart distinct flavors and can contribute to the color and moisture of the crust.
- **Diabetic Friendly:** For a lower glycemic index, consider using natural sweeteners like coconut sugar or agave syrup, which are processed more slowly by the body than regular sugar.

5. Increase Vegetable Content:
- **Vegetable Purees:** Integrate vegetable purees such as pumpkin, sweet potato, or beetroot into your dough. These not only add moisture and natural sweetness but are also packed with vitamins.
- **Leafy Greens:** Finely chopped or pureed greens like spinach or kale can be mixed into the dough for an extra dose of nutrients without altering the bread's texture significantly.

6. Enhance with Fermentation:
- **Longer Fermentation:** Extending the fermentation period allows for a greater breakdown of phytates, which improves mineral absorption and adds to the depth of flavor in your sourdough.
- **Sourdough Efficiency:** The natural fermentation process in sourdough helps to pre-digest gluten and starches, making the bread easier to digest and nutrients more accessible.

By integrating these tips into your sourdough baking, you not only create healthier bread but also enrich the culinary experience with new flavors and textures. These nutritional enhancements make sourdough an even more valuable addition to a balanced diet, allowing you to enjoy your baking creations with added health benefits.

BONUS MEAL PLAN

Important Notes:

- **Customization is Key:** Adjust portion sizes and ingredients to fit your individual needs and preferences.
- **Hydration Matters:** Don't forget to drink plenty of water throughout the day!
- **Leftovers are Your Friend:** Cook larger batches and incorporate leftovers into other meals to save time and avoid food waste.
- **Listen to Your Body:** It's okay to have treats or higher-calorie days occasionally – balance is key to a sustainable diet.

Here's a sample meal plan structure. Keep in mind that you can substitute any of your fabulous recipes throughout the 30 days to add variety!

Meal Plan Structure

Day	Breakfast	Lunch	Snacks	Dinner
Day 1	Almond Berry Burst Muffin + Greek yogurt	Tropical Twist Panzanella + hard-boiled egg	1/2 apple + handful of nuts	Shrimp & Avocado Delight Sourdough Pizza

Day	Breakfast	Lunch	Snacks	Dinner
Day 2	Protein-Packed Pumpkin Power Pancakes	Lentil & Mushroom Stuffing with a mixed green salad	Banana Chia Bites	Spiced Lentil & Quinoa Sourdough Bagel + veggie sticks
Day 3	Sunrise Surprise Muffin + Berries	Quinoa, Kale & Cranberry Stuffing + grilled chicken breast	Spiced Carrot & Raisin Biscuits	Mediterranean Feast Sourdough Pizza
Day 4	Fluffy Banana & Greek Yogurt Pancakes	Savory Protein Kick Muffin + Carrot sticks	1/2 pear + Nutty Chocolate Chip Cookies (1-2)	Thai-Inspired Chicken Sourdough Pizza
Day 5	Chia Seed Powerhouse Muffins	Mediterranean Olive & Feta Crumble Crostini Salad	Blueberry Lemon Zest Cookies (1-2)	Lentil & Veggie Lover's Sourdough Pizza
Day 6	Savory Ricotta & Herb Waffles	Greek-inspired Panzanella + sliced grilled chicken or tofu	1/2 cup mixed berries + Tropical Coconut Bites (1-2)	Chicken & Herb Sourdough Biscuits + Roasted vegetables (broccoli, carrots, asparagus)
Day 7	Carrot Cake Fusion Pancakes + fruit	Chickpea & Herb Surprise Crackers with veggie sticks	Banana with peanut butter	Lentil & Veggie Lover's Sourdough Pizza
Day 8	Protein Power Bagel + cream cheese & smoked salmon	Mediterranean Panzanella + hard-boiled egg	Handful of mixed nuts	Spiced Lentil & Quinoa Stuffed Peppers

Day	Breakfast	Lunch	Snacks	Dinner
Day 9	Nutty Pear Spice Muffin + Greek Yogurt	Leftover Stuffed Peppers	1/2 cup mixed berries + Tropical Coconut Bites (1-2)	Thai-Inspired Chicken Sourdough Pizza
Day 10	Chocolate Avocado Delight Muffin	Southwestern Black Bean & Corn Salad + Sourdough Croutons	Apple slices + Nutty Chocolate Chip Cookies (1-2)	Sourdough Bagel Sandwich (turkey, cheese, pesto)
Day 11	Almond Berry Burst Muffin	Roasted Red Pepper & Feta Dip with Seeded Crackers & veggies	1/2 pear with almond butter	Shrimp & Avocado Delight Sourdough Pizza
Day 12	Savory Ricotta & Herb Waffles	Quinoa, Kale & Cranberry Stuffing + grilled tofu	A handful of trail mix	Lentil & Mushroom Stuffing + Roasted Vegetables
Day 13	Sunrise Surprise Muffin + Berries	Mediterranean Olive & Feta Crumble Crostini Salad	Banana Chia Bites	Spicy Chorizo & Pineapple Sourdough Pizza
Day 14	Fluffy Banana & Greek Yogurt Pancakes	Greek-Inspired Panzanella + Grilled Chicken	Oatmeal Apricot Power Cookies (1-2)	Chicken & Herb Sourdough Biscuits + side salad

Day	Breakfast	Lunch	Snacks	Dinner
Day 15	Tropical Chia Powerhouse Muffin	Black Bean & Corn Salad with Avocado & Lime Vinaigrette + Crackers	Spiced Carrot & Raisin Cookies (1-2)	Sourdough Bagel Sandwich (hummus, roasted veggies, sprouts)
Day 16	Kiwi Chia Burst Pancakes	Lentil & Mushroom Stuffing with a mixed green salad	Spiced Carrot & Raisin Biscuits (1-2)	Mediterranean Feast Sourdough Pizza
Day 17	Savory Protein Kick Muffin + Berries	Quinoa & Avocado Hummus with Pita Bread & Carrot sticks	Apple with Sunflower Seed Butter	Stuffed Zucchini Boats (ground turkey, rice, sourdough breadcrumbs, tomato sauce)
Day 18	Protein-Packed Pumpkin Power Pancakes	Leftover Stuffed Zucchini Boats	Handful of mixed nuts	Thai-Inspired Chicken Sourdough Pizza
Day 19	Raspberry & Quinoa Power Muffin + Greek Yogurt	Spinach & Artichoke Dip with Everything Bagel Crostini & veggies	1/2 pear with Nutty Chocolate Chip Cookies (1-2)	Lentil & Veggie Lover's Sourdough Pizza
Day 20	Jackfruit & Coconut Surprise Pancakes	White Bean & Spinach Spread on Sourdough Bread + Salad	Oatmeal Apricot Power Cookies (1-2)	Sourdough Bagel Sandwich (Tuna salad, lettuce, tomato)

Day	Breakfast	Lunch	Snacks	Dinner
Day 21	Blueberry Lemon Zest Muffin	Leftover tuna salad with Seeded Powerhouse Crackers	Fruit with Yogurt & Granola (use sourdough breadcrumbs)	Shrimp & Avocado Delight Sourdough Pizza
Day 22	Tropical Chia Powerhouse Muffin (Repeat)	Roasted Red Pepper & Feta Dip with Everything Bagel Crostini & veggies	Banana Chia Bites	Chicken & Herb Sourdough Biscuits + Roasted Vegetables
Day 23	Nutty Pear Spice Muffin	Greek-Inspired Panzanella + grilled tofu	Handful of almonds and dried cranberries	Spiced Lentil & Quinoa Stuffed Peppers (Repeat)
Day 24	Savory Ricotta & Herb Waffles	Cream of Carrot & Quinoa Soup + Sourdough Croutons	Apple slices with peanut butter	Sourdough Pizza (Experiment with creative toppings!)
Day 25	Carrot Cake Fusion Pancakes (Repeat)	Black Bean & Corn Salad + Avocado & Lime Vinaigrette + Crackers	Banana with Sunflower Seed Butter	Lentil & Mushroom Stuffing with a Side Salad
Day 26	Choose a Favorite Muffin	Leftover pizza (reheat or repurpose toppings)	Fruit with yogurt & sourdough granola	Curried Chickpeas & Vegetables with Sourdough Naan or Flatbread

Day	Breakfast	Lunch	Snacks	Dinner
Day 27	Pancakes (Repeat a winner)	Big Salad - Base of quinoa/lentils, grilled protein of choice, leftover roasted veggies, sourdough croutons, favorite dressing	Handful of nuts & dried fruit	Sourdough Bagel Sandwich (creative combo!)
Day 28	Savory Waffles or Biscuits	Mediterranean Panzanella (use leftover grilled protein or chickpeas)	Spiced Carrot & Raisin Cookies (1-2)	Stuffed Peppers or Zucchini Boats (if you didn't tire of them earlier!)
Day 29	Breakfast of Choice (Repeat or try a new combo)	A large batch of favorite soup + sourdough bread/crackers	Banana Chia Bites or other snack favorite	A Comfort Food Twist: Mac & Cheese with sourdough breadcrumbs or a casserole with a sourdough base
Day 30	Celebration Breakfast: Choose a special muffin or pancake recipe	Leftovers turned into a creative, colorful salad	Pick your favorite snack	Final Sourdough Pizza Night - go all out with toppings!

About The Author

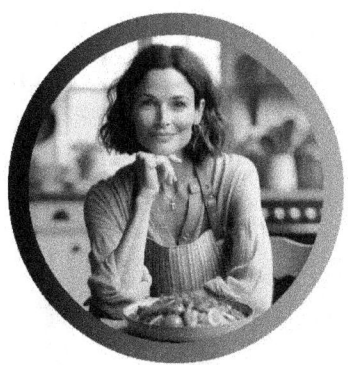

Samantha Bax, an advocate of vegan, eco-mindful cuisine, discovered her true passion in the heart of a bustling city. However, her culinary journey didn't start in a kitchen but rather in her grandmother's cozy home, where she first learned the importance of nourishing and wholesome eating.

When Samantha was diagnosed with diabetes during her twenties, her life took a turn. This pivotal moment fueled her commitment to health and well-being, leading her to become a certified nutritionist. Fate had something in store for Samantha when a close family member was diagnosed with kidney disease. This significant event brought together her two passions. Food and wellness. Inspiring her to create a niche that caters to both renal diets.

Course Samantha faced challenges along the way. Balancing health requirements while maintaining flavors proved to be quite complex. However, she remained steadfast in refusing to compromise taste for the sake of health. To overcome this obstacle, Samantha embarked on an adventure where she sought inspiration from kitchens across the Mediterranean region, vibrant spice markets in Asia, and sustainable farms throughout Central America.

In **"Gluten-Free Sourdough Bread Recipes for Beginners"** Samantha Bax beautifully intertwines her story with an enticing collection of mouth-watering recipes.

She strongly believes that food is not a means of survival. Also, it is something to be cherished as a way to celebrate life and promote well-being.

The main aim of her book is to present readers with a curated collection of recipes that cater to their needs while also providing them with an enjoyable culinary experience.

Apart from writing and experimenting in the kitchen, Samantha finds joy in the art of photography. She skillfully captures the essence of cityscapes, as well as serene landscapes, in nature. Furthermore, she actively leads workshops and seminars where she guides individuals on how to make food choices that prioritize taste without compromising on quality.

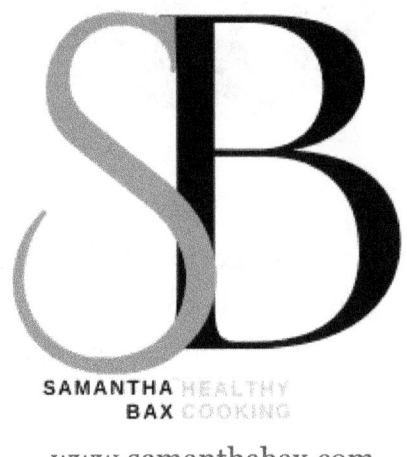

www.samanthabax.com

To join our Newsletter and receive advance notification of new publications, subscribe to the Newsletter for FREE today at:

www.prosebooks.com/subscribe

Other Books By Samantha Bax

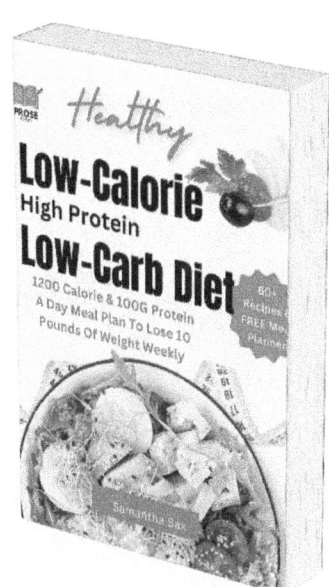
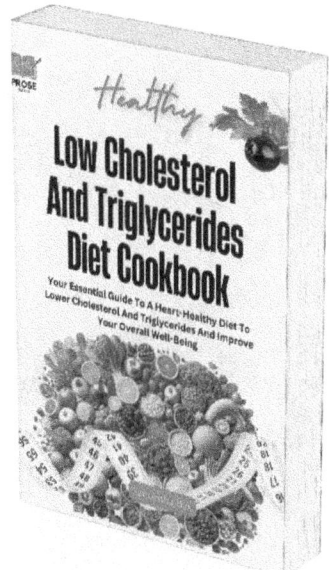
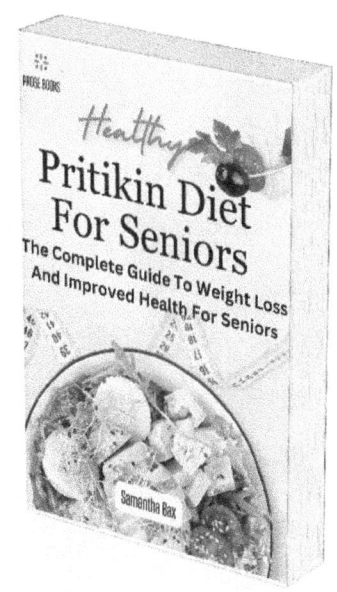
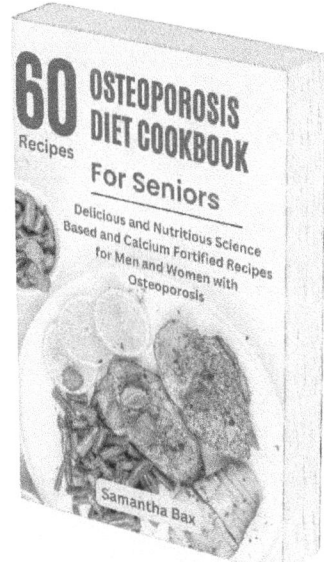
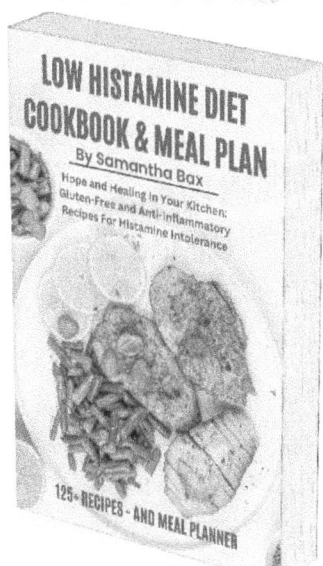
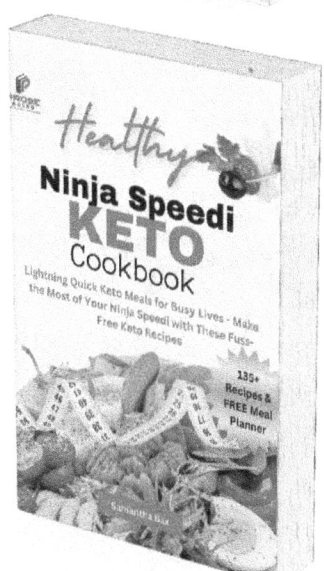

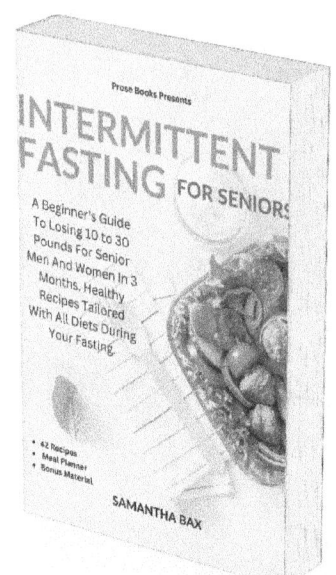
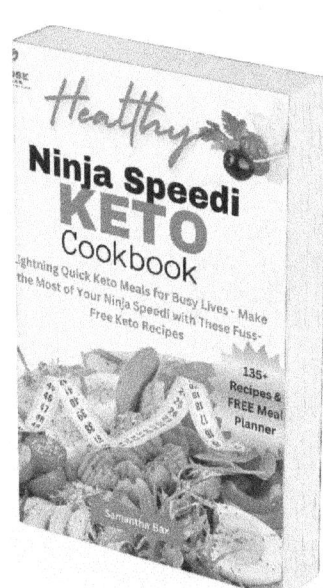
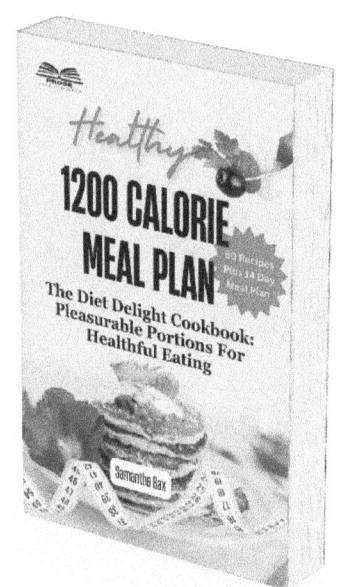
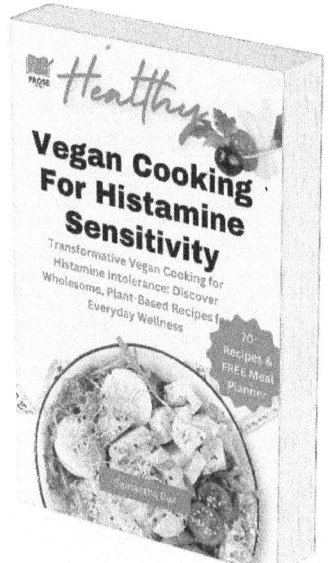
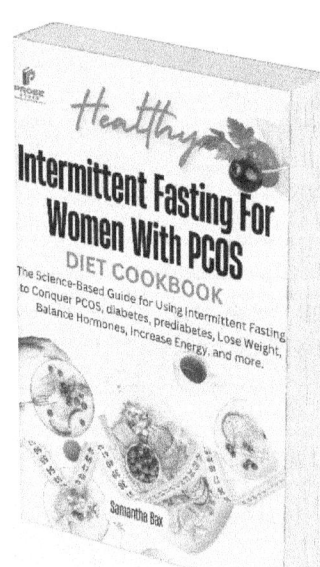
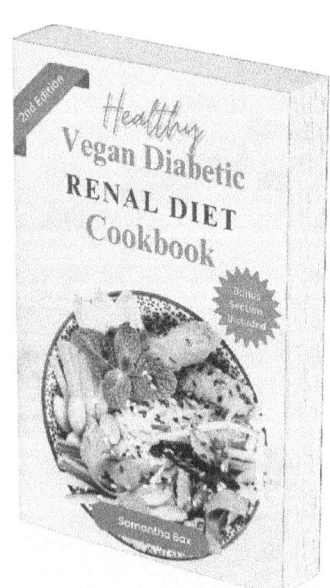

Scan the above code to see all of the books and more...
https://shop.prosebooks.com

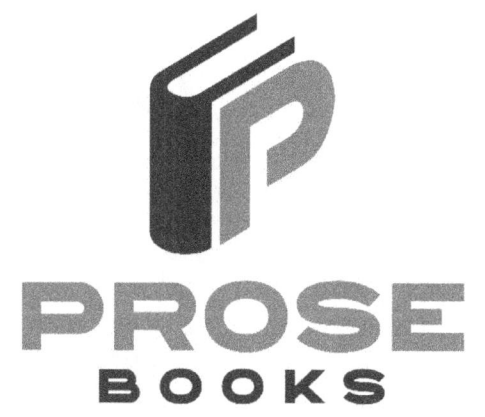

Empowering Authors, Forging Legacies

Thank You

Dear Reader,

As we approach the end of this journey, I want to express my sincere gratitude to you for embracing these recipes in your kitchen and, in turn, in your life. Your support means the world to me. It ignites my passion for sharing the goodness that food brings to our tables and our souls.

May the flavors you've explored and the nourishment you've derived from these pages inspire moments of happiness, connection, and well-being. Always remember that every meal you prepare is an expression of your imagination and thoughtfulness.

Looking forward to our escapade,

Warmest regards,

Samantha Bax

BONUS: FREE Meal-Planner

As a FREE Bonus to all my readers, I invite you to go to my publisher's website at www.prosebooks.com/meal-planner and get a FREE Meal Planner to help and guide you along your journey to fitness and good health.

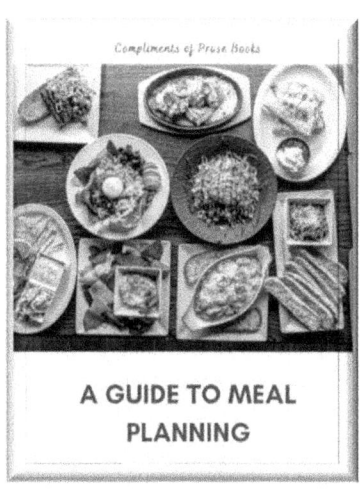

www.ingramcontent.com/pod-product-compliance
Lightning Source LLC
Chambersburg PA
CBHW080439110426
42743CB00016B/3213